101 Helps for Helpers

by

DR. LINDA JOHNSON CROWELL

with
FOREWORD BY BISHOP JONATHAN D. KEATON
FOREWORD BY REV. DR. JULIUS C. TRIMBLE
EDITORIAL ASSISTANCE BY MARK R. CROWELL

authorHOUSE®

AuthorHouse™
1663 Liberty Drive, Suite 200
Bloomington, IN 47403
www.authorhouse.com
Phone: 1-800-839-8640

First published by AuthorHouse 4/14/2009

ISBN: 978-1-4343-5601-7 (sc)
ISBN: 978-1-4343-5602-4 (hc)

Library of Congress Control Number: 2007909727

Printed in the United States of America
Bloomington, Indiana

This book is printed on acid-free paper.

Dedication

WHEN I THINK of those persons who have influenced and inspired me as I have traveled the road of life, I must first and foremost thank God for my parents, Albert and Naomi Johnson. Although they have ended their earthly journeys, they continue to live in the lessons they taught and the ways they tried to help others. They were always giving of themselves and sharing of the meager yet bountiful resources they had through their hard work and God's provision. They taught their seven children to love God, to love ourselves, to love our fellow humans, and to show that love in acts of kindness to others.

Consequently, I must also dedicate this book to my siblings who continue to embody what our parents taught us: Betty Jackson, Jeanette Johnson, Rosetta Hall, Albert Johnson, Jr., Dianne East, and Charlene Benn. Many of the stories shared in the book and many of the special times that have brought delight to my life emanate from the blessings of a happy and joyful childhood. My days are filled with cherished memories of family times together, family sharing, and a family network of love and support. When I think of our rich heritage of reflecting Jesus through acts of helping and caring, I pray that this will be the legacy we leave to our children for generations to come.

I also thank my husband, Henry Crowell, who always supports my endeavors, and our son, Mark Crowell who urges me on and provides technical assistance for my writings and other endeavors such as the Helpfullsource. com website and Help-Full Source Ministry.

Finally, I must thank my social work students. After nearly twenty years as a social worker, I joined the faculty of the University of Akron (Ohio) School of Social Work. Eleven years on the faculty provided many opportunities to instruct and impact the lives of continuing and aspiring social workers from the University of Akron and Cleveland (Ohio) State University. As I reflect on my many conversations and interactions with students, I recall hearing of their struggles to provide the best service to those they served, often with meager resources and feeling unappreciated. They were balancing many priorities and often I would get last minute calls that a student could not make class because of an "emergency situation" with a client. As I thought of some way to provide support and inspiration to my students, the idea of this book took root. And it is with the prayer that this book will be a resource and a source of spiritual grounding that I say, "Thank you students for providing me with impetus to begin the book. I hope this book will serve as a tool that you will find useful as you move along in your helping journey."

Foreword

Bishop Jonathan D. Keaton

IN THE GENRE of *The Upper Room* and *The Daily Word*, native Georgian, Linda Johnson Crowell writes, ruminates, remembers, and rejoices. Daily life and childhood years, Scripture and God are the main portals for her narratives. Some of her reflections are theological. Others are practical. Still other narratives recount trips abroad where God came alive in the worship and spirit of the people of Africa, or in Mexico where faith in God taught important lessons.

To be sure the pithy meditations in the Crowell text are for devotional purposes. Yet, they are something more. Her meditations can function as gateways to Bible study, introspective journaling, or face-to-face discussion groups. They can inspire sermon topics and thus provide rich illustrations to entice the listening audience. These meditations can provide relevant grist for chat room conversations; they cause one to want to explore the Scriptures more, to go more deeply into discussion and discourse that emanate from the catchy titles. More importantly, the work itself serves as a reminder to persons of the Christian faith. To know what we believe, to embrace what we believe, to converse and struggle with what we believe, biblical, theological, and life experiences require the best inquiry and commitment we can give to study and exploration of God's word.

Many are burdened with the tasks of helping others, often with no outlet or spiritual resource geared to their needs. *101 Helps for Helpers* is a good primer on "being there for God." This book provides inspiration relevant to different ways we help and care for others. It incorporates the many realties that helpers and caregivers face. It provides refreshment for the many who manifest Jesus by being there for others—for so many who take on roles of caring for others. *Taste and See.*

Bishop Jonathan D. Keaton
Resident Bishop Michigan Area
United Methodist Church

Foreword

Rev. Dr. Julius C. Trimble

I HAVE SOME very good news to share. Many people are going to be blessed by this insightful book. Many will cherish this book and refer to it for years to come. Many will share the blessings of this book whose time has come with others. In her first publication, Dr. Linda Johnson Crowell offers readers a treasure trove of encouragement using daily devotions that come alive with inspiration. Rooted in Scripture from the Old and New Testaments, these daily meditations are relevant as they challenge and comfort.

We are invited into the rich personal experiences of Linda and her family as we latch onto many moments that are so much a part of the universal experience of the human family. As readers we are fortified in our faith as hope and joy themes are presented in digestible bites.

If you have wanted for a long time to read the Bible in a disciplined and devotional way, this book is for you. If you like me choose to begin or end your day with a devotional reading, this book is the ticket. As a preacher who is always looking for help with sermon material and solid sources, I am shouting hallelujah! Dr. Linda Crowell has done a great service in sharing her insights in such a way that preachers of the Gospel and teachers of the Bible can be rewarded with stories that most people can relate to. Daily devotional books are not a new phenomenon. However, the combination of prose, poetry, and a *Nugget for Today* provides a fresh breath of spiritual encouragement needed for the stress and mess that is so much a part of Twenty-First Century living.

By way of example three of the daily offerings gave me insight into the author's gift of making deep and theologically important points enjoyably understandable. *Ric-Rac Joy (about staying connected)*, gives personal insight into one of Jesus' foundational messages on the vine and branches. Using her childhood experience of the *Ric-Rac or Paddle Ball toy*, the reader is encouraged to stay connected to Jesus and others. *Boomerang Joy and A Drop in the Bucket* illustrate Dr. Linda Crowell's stewardship of words that capture the reader's interest. In a wonderful story from Charleston, South Carolina we are encouraged by the testimony of one who lives a simple life and gives so much to bless others. As we give, the joy of giving returns as a blessing—just like a *boomerang*.

The importance of one is captured in a profound way in *A Drop in the Bucket*. Every soul, every person, every child, lost or found is important to God. Jesus' teaching from Luke 15 comes alive in a way that invites us to celebrate the small successes and often overlooked miracles of life. Dr. Linda Crowell applies modern-day titles and phrases such as "emergency preparedness" and "cruise control" to illustrate how Scripture is as relevant today as when it was first recorded.

Before I became her pastor in 2003, I knew Dr. Linda Crowell as a Christian woman who had much to offer the world by way of her living witness. As an active teacher, social worker, researcher, and inspirational speaker, she has mentored students and encouraged countless others with her gift of Christian insight and spiritual encouragement. As an active leader at Aldersgate United Methodist Church, Linda has taught Women's Bible Study classes and led our Church Council with a sensitivity to the priority of "worshipful work" and "can do spirit."

The fall of 2006 I joined Dr. Linda Crowell and five other leaders from the East Ohio Conference of the United Methodist Church on an advance mission trip to West Africa. In Liberia and Sierra Leone we met many people and traveled to rural villages to observe health clinics and schools. Linda took detailed notes but always put away pen and paper to be fully present with the people in the moment. A global citizen who is unapologetically Christian, on one occasion she spoke to women in Liberia and said, " I am one of you, one with you." This sensitivity to God's gift of the present moment comes through clearly in this book for all God's people.

Thank you Linda Crowell. God has used you to make a difference with the gift of pen and prayer. May all who read this book be encouraged daily. Help has arrived! Take out your Bibles, a journal, and a pen, and reflect on these rich offerings for the journey.

Rev. Dr. Julius C. Trimble, Pastor
Aldersgate United Methodist Church
Warrensville Heights, Ohio

Introduction

Why This Book?
Dr. Linda Johnson Crowell

HELPS FOR THE helper. Helpers you are not alone. Who is a helper you ask? Well, I believe every human being was created to be a helper. After God created man, Adam, He created, Eve, woman, to be a "help-meet"—one who helps (Genesis 2:18). We first see that Cain, who after killing his brother, Abel sensed that God had created humans to care for each other when he asked God, "Am I my brother's keeper?" (Genesis 4:9). Yes, I believe we all were created to be our sisters' and brothers' keepers and helpers as Paul tells the Galatians, "Bear one another's burdens and so fulfill the law of Christ" (Galatians 6:2). And so, I exhort helpers and caregivers to use spiritual encouragement as you embody what God has created you to be. In Ephesians 4:12, we find that God prepared "some people for works of service." So, live a life worthy of your calling. And further, we are all helpers as we are told to encourage one another and build each other up (I Thessalonians 5:11).

In Acts 9:36 we find Tabitha, a helper for she was "always doing good and helping the poor." The Bible again tells us that there are "those able to help others" (1 Corinthians 12:28), further affirming the fact that God has equipped some to be helpers. God also speaks of a reward. We can be assured by these words from Colossians 3:23, "Whatever you do, work at it with all your heart, as working for the Lord, not men." Yes this is our job description; and as a reward or bonus for our service, helpers will "receive an inheritance from the Lord as a reward." All of us should be helpers in some way.

And so, "Let us clothe ourselves with compassion, kindness, humility, gentleness, and patience" (Colossians 3:12). These qualities should define our demeanor. And, let us endeavor each day to: "be joyful always, pray continually; give thanks in all circumstances, for this is God's will for you in Christ Jesus" (1 Thessalonians 5:16). These things define our spiritual grounding. Helpers and caregivers, I pray God will give you strength for your journey.

It is my hope that the catchy titles will peak your interest to anticipate how the **Verse for Today** relates to the title. It is my hope that the daily meditation will cause you to smile, laugh, reflect on your own experiences, and create your own stories of the rhythm of life as you make the connection between Scripture and life. It is my hope that the **meditation for the day** will lift your spirits, give you new insights, and serve as a spiritual resource. It is my hope that these messages will affirm the importance of being a helper and caregiver. It is my hope that the **Nugget for Today** will give you something to ground and energize you, and give you something to focus on each day.

Most importantly, it is my prayer that the **Prayer for Today** will connect you to the God who hears your prayers and grants your requests in His time, in His way, according to His will, for you and on behalf of others. You will notice that each prayer except the final one ends without an Amen. This is to encourage continuous prayers as you navigate each day, hoping you will add to the prayer as trying situations arise, and that you may offer prayers of thanksgiving as you see joy, triumphs, and breakthroughs. Prayers are in the plural form. It is my prayer that as many helpers and caregivers are praying the same prayer that we will be a group of intercessors on behalf all helpers and those we help.

I hope you will find many ways to use this book and that you will share it with others. I hope you use it as a source of daily meditation, that you will use it to guide your journaling, and that you will use it to delve deeper into the Bible. I also hope you will be inspired to collect your own stories, begin your own writings, and use this experience to further enhance your spiritual growth and affirmation of being in service to others—you are a helper.

Dr. Linda Johnson Crowell

Contents

YOU-Nique

VERSE FOR TODAY: Psalm 139:13-14

For you created my inmost being; you knit me together in my mother's womb. I praise you, because I am fearfully and wonderfully made; your works are wonderful.

THE *NELSON'S NEW King James Study Bible* uses the phrase, "I am fearfully and wonderfully made." This might also be rephrased as, "I am an awesome wonder." Oh to think that before you were even born, Elohim God, the Great Creator had already set the universe in place to accommodate and honor the occasion of your birth. Before your mother was even born, before she conceived you, God had ordained your birth, who your parents would be, when and where you would be born, and the circumstances of your birth. God, with His wisdom and vision, had already set in motion the physical characteristics for the special creation you would be, even down to the "number of hairs on your head" (Matthew 10:30).

If you reflect on your date of birth, millions of other people around the world were born at the exact time that you were. However, none of them is a replication or duplication of you. Even if you are an identical twin in man's view, you are a *YOU-nique* creation of God. No other person has your special set of genes, personality, or make-up. In man's best attempts, he has made strides toward manipulating the birth process, even so far as to create "test tube babies" and involving other means of tampering with conception and birth. Nevertheless, every person and soul has God's stamp for God's divine plan.

Psalm 8:4 asks: "What is man that you are mindful of him; and the son of man that you visit him?" Ask yourself, why did God endow you with the qualities that enable you to help others and care for others? Why were you chosen to minister to others and help others live the life God intended? Even before creation, God knew that you would follow the path to help others and care for others; therefore since God has crowned man (you) with glory and honor (Psalm 8: 5) use your *YOU-niqueness* to make a difference today. As the psalmist says in the beginning and end of Psalm 8, "O Lord, Our Lord, How majestic is your name in all the earth!" How thoughtful of Great Creator God to put the stamp of approval on people like you to be in the ministry of helping and caring for others.

Nugget for Today: I am an awesome wonder.

Prayer for Today: Dear God, we thank You that we are fearfully and wonderfully made. How divinely perceptive of You to create and ordain persons who even without their planning it, would be a source of help, healing, and hope for others. Lord, You have placed us in the role of helping others and caring for others. Each day is a struggle between knowing the best way to make a difference in the lives of so many suffering people and so many who don't know to call on You as Lord and Savior. Often we find ourselves questioning why some people seem to always be in need of help and guidance to meet even their basic needs, and why some never get out of the rut of barely surviving day-to-day. But we know that You have stamped everyone with Your divine plan, and we pray that we will be strengthened to use our *YOU-niqueness* to make a difference in the lives of others...

Re-Joy-SING

Sing to the LORD, all the earth; proclaim his salvation day after day.

SINGING AND RE-"JOY-SING" are presented in so many places in the Bible, especially the book of Psalms. Psalm 81 begins with: "Sing for joy to God to God our strength." In fact, the call to sing or the act of singing can be found in numerous passages in the Old Testament, and several times in the New Testament. In Acts 16:25 we find Paul and Silas praying and singing hymns to God and the other prisoners were listening to them. They were *re-joy-SING* even while in prison. James 5: 13 offers singing as part of what many helpers call a treatment plan. James provides the following action steps: *"Is anyone among you suffering? Let him pray. Is anyone cheerful, let him sing Psalms"* (New King James Version). Praying and singing—a divine prescription.

Have you ever awakened during the night or faced the dawn of a new day with a song in your heart? For quite some time I was unaware of songs that infused my being some days. By happenstance, or should I say by Divine Inspiration, one day I became keenly aware that during some nights and early mornings, I was being awakened with a song. For a spell, I kept a record of these songs. In my subconscious, I was being given a song to help me face the challenge of the day and days to come, or a song of joy and celebration for blessings and triumphs. Some of the words and titles were: *Your grace and mercy; Jesus build a fence all around me every day; I need you, you need me; come on in where the table is set; no weapon formed against me; O Lord, how excellent is your name, there is none like You; Jesus, you're the center of my joy; is your all on the altar?; I got the love of Jesus down in my soul; when there's nothing left but God, that's all you need; God is a wonder to my soul;* and among my favorites: *Order My Steps in Your Word.*

Perhaps you have been aware of the songs of your subconscious, or perhaps this is a time to listen for a special song from God. I believe that it is hard to sing and not end up *re-joy-SING*, even when the weight of the world seems upon you. So, don't fight it, sing with all your might, and even break free in a dance as David did—close the doors of your office, do a "car dance" while in traffic, use the aisles in the sanctuary, "begin the music, strike the tambourine, play the melodious harp and lyre …" (Psalm 81: 2). Everyone has some reason for re-Joy-SING!

NUGGET FOR TODAY: I will spend some time each day *re-joy-SING*!

PRAYER FOR TODAY: Dear Lord, You gave us the gift of music and the ability to sing. We may feel we lack angelic voices, but You always stand ready to listen to our feeble attempts to sing praises. You put a song in our hearts if we would just listen for it. Help us to find some reason to sing each day and help us to sing our way through those rough days. Infuse us with words and melodies what will make each thing we experience focus on You and rejoice in You. Help us to inspire those we will be helping and caring for today to find some small reason to sing; and even give them healing words and special reasons to sing. Help us to spread the Good News; help us to help others to find their special song. We pray for the energy to spend precious time today in the spirit of *re-joy-SING!...*

Miserable Is For Someone Else

VERSE FOR TODAY: Job 2:10

Shall we accept good from God, and not trouble?

THIS WAS JOB'S response after earlier having lost his property and his children. At this point in his loss, Job was stricken with boils that left no part of his body untouched. Sitting in the midst of desolation, Job used a potsherd (or piece of broken pottery) to scrape away the scabs of these painful growths. Festering boils had been described earlier in Exodus as one of the plagues that befell the Egyptians when they refused to release the Israelites from bondage (Exodus 9:9-11). They sound awful.

Seeing his detestable physical appearance, Job's wife advised him to "curse God and die" (Job 2:9). But Job refused to follow her advice and he refused to wallow in misery. Job gave a response that continues to resonate with me when I see hard times. His response: "Shall we accept good from God and not trouble?" Job 2:10 is one verse that can aid helpers, their clients, patients, parishioners, loved ones, and persons they care for to transcend current situations and find hope and inspiration in all that Job experienced.

Public policy continues to erode away the already fragile "safety nets" for children, the poor, the elderly, and the disenfranchised. The growing push for euthanasia and assisted suicide points to modern-day intolerance for pain, suffering, and despair. The increase in the suicide rates is involving our youth in staggering numbers—further pointing to our intolerance for physical as well as mental, and emotional misery or discomfort. But through all his trials, Job refused to be miserable. Sitting among the ruins and ashes, Job tried to scrape away the physical pain; but he kept the faith. His response challenges us to trust God during the good and the bad times. Why bad things happen to good people is the pervasive theme of the book of Job and is a question that many helpers and caregivers ask about the suffering they see.

Job exemplified a stance that led him to leave the misery to someone else. He held steadfast to the promise of a better tomorrow. When Job needed his wife the most, she accused him of holding on to his integrity (Job 2:9); and she let him down. She thought Job's religious beliefs had gone so far that he refused to accept reality, when in essence his religion was just beginning to "kick in!" His faith allowed him to counter his accusers with his blamelessness. He chastised and admonished them with steadfast words: *"Though he slay me, yet I will hope in him..."* (Job 13:15).

NUGGET FOR TODAY: **I refuse to be miserable today.**

PRAYER FOR TODAY: Dear Loving and Steadfast God, though You slay us, we will still hope in You. We pray that we can communicate Your goodness and Your mercy to those we come in contact with today. Let us <u>not</u> be like Job's wife, by giving curt words without understanding the way You, our Great God operates. Let us <u>not</u> be like Job's friends who were judgmental and accusatory refusing to believe in Job's righteousness. May we <u>not</u> be so preoccupied with possessions and worldly things that we make ourselves miserable without them. Help us to stand firm in the face of illness, pain, and adversity; help us to teach those we help today how to accept both misery and goodness from You. Help us to know when to listen; teach us how to hear the needs of others. Guide the words that we speak. May they be words of comfort; may they <u>not</u> stem from piety or self-conceit. And even though we cannot explain suffering, help us to find words of comfort and assurance and help others to **refuse to be miserable...**

Take A Joy Pit Stop

VERSE FOR TODAY: 1 Thessalonians 1:6

You became imitators [followers] of us and of the Lord; in spite of severe suffering, you welcomed the message with the joy given by the Holy Spirit.

AS IN A race, sometimes it's necessary to take a pit stop. Just as a racecar needs gas, a change of tires, new engines, and repairs, so does the helper. When the checkered flag is waved, racecars get off to a record-breaking start, in full throttle, aimed at the finish line. Is this how you start your day?

The Thessalonians received the gospel in an environment of persecution. Nonetheless, they received the Word with the joy of the Holy Spirit. A race seems to be the day-to-day setting for many in the helping professions. The race is grueling; crashes can occur at any second; tires can blow out at any minute; the driver can misjudge a curve. Sometimes a driver may be involved in an accident or has to leave the race because of the actions of another driver-akin to the pressure and derailment felt by many helpers. Clients', patients', and parishioners' lives may be mostly impacted by the actions of others-their lives are derailed by someone in the next lane. Even helpers receive backlash, admonishment, criticism—crashes despite their best actions and intentions.

Maybe we should learn from Paul. Paul knew how to take joy pit stops. He found ways to use his pit crew. He looked for joy in all the right places. For example, he found joy in the report he received from his young protégé, Titus, about the progress the Corinthians were making. He rejoiced even more over their mourning and repentance (2 Corinthians 7:9). Again, he rejoiced for the joy of Titus (2 Corinthians 7:6). In addition, he rejoiced over the Macedonians who gave generously during their afflictions, in spite of their poverty. They gave with great joy (2 Corinthians 8:2).

As Paul took pit stops to change the tires and refuel his joy during his race, so must the helper. With the Holy Spirit and Jesus as the heads of the pit crew, Paul found the fuel needed to face his tribulations, trials and suffering, criticism, and even his mysterious "thorn in the flesh" (2 Corinthians12:7).

Using Paul as an example, we can go to the Source of the fuel and fill our tanks with much needed joy. We don't even have to worry about rising gas prices. As our clients make progress, our patients heal, and our congregations develop a deeper relationship with God, we can be refreshed despite the persecution and condemnation that an uncaring world throws at helpers and those we serve. We can get regular fill-ups of joy.

NUGGET FOR TODAY: **I will make regular joy pit stops.**

PRAYER FOR TODAY: Dear Source of all power and fuel, help us to know when we need a change of tires or a fill-up. Help us to find things to rejoice over and to find things to keep us focused on filling ourselves and directing others to Your fill-up station. Help us find joy in those we meet along the way such as the Thessalonians, the Corinthians, and the Macedonians—those who make changes with mourning and repentance, who give generously despite their poverty, and those young persons you put in our lives who need mentoring and support. Lord, help us to persevere despite any afflictions we may have; help us to be refreshed as we race around a seemingly endless track; help us to be confident to pull up to the tank, fill up to the brim, and find the fuel and joy that are offered through Christ Jesus and the Holy Spirit...

My Niece's Cat

VERSE FOR TODAY: Exodus 31:15

For six days, work is to be done, but the seventh day is a Sabbath of rest, holy to the LORD.

MY FAMILY ENGAGES in spirited, joyful, full-of-laughter conference calls every Sunday night. The seven of us use this as a time of catching up on news, discussing the highlights of the day's church services, discussing sermons by our Sister, Rev. Dr. Betty Jackson, giving praise reports, and taking care of family business. We also talk on holidays. Last Christmas, my sister informed us they had a new family member. We were all curious. Well Kaci the cat was my niece Peyton's Christmas present.

In all honesty, I was not too thrilled about the idea of a cat. I admit I don't have an instant affection for cats. Something about them makes me uneasy. I thought I may never visit my sister again—Kaci ruled the house it seemed. Well, I bit the bullet and stayed with them while I was attending a conference in Atlanta. I braced myself for Kaci, who immediately came to inspect me. She sniffed everything about me. I put my things in the guest bedroom and closed the door—my mental sign saying "Keep Out Kaci." Kaci has a bell around her neck. So I knew where she was at all times. She was everywhere at all times with the bell ringing as she roamed the house.

My sister and nieces went away for a while. Another niece and a nephew came to keep me company. They began to run around the family room hundreds of times with Kaci chasing after a cat toy. All of a sudden, Kaci stopped in the middle of the floor, laid down, looked around, and immediately went to sleep on her back with her feet in the air. I panicked. I thought she had run herself to death. She didn't seem to be breathing. I kept asking, "Is Kaci all right?" My niece and nephew who should have taken a cue from Kaci said, "Sure, she does that when she gets tired—she stops and takes a nap."

Well, I could have used a nap by then. I was tired from the trip, worn out from laughing and reminiscing with my family, and tired out from seeing them run around. And so I thought: "If Kaci has enough sense to rest, why don't we?" Yes, I realize Kaci doesn't have a job, or spouse, or children, or others to care for, or the hassles we humans have; but, a good rest or "power nap" would give us the energy to spring to life again like Kaci did after a few minutes, and start the *rat race* all over again. Just as we awoke from our naps at nursery school with renewed energy, a "siesta" would do us all good.

Years back, I aspired to see how much vacation time I could accumulate. As I wound down my working years, I tried to make sure to use all the time I had accumulated. Rest is necessary to deal with the daily hassles. Like Kaci, may helpers and caregivers find more seasons of rest and respite—waking up refreshed to help even more.

Nugget for Today: Like Kaci, I will take time to rest.

Prayer for Today: Dear God and Creator of Rest, may we be mindful of your Word and may we take cues from Your creations to stop and rest. We may not be able to just stop and go to sleep like Kaci, but we know You will provide opportunities for "time outs." Help us to take advantage of the times provided for breaks, vacation time, personal days, retreats. Help us to get away from the "rat race" to find peace and quiet. Give us seasons of refreshment and energy to rebound. May we be like those in many countries who structure time for "siestas." Help us be attuned to our bodies and the messages You give us to slow down, lie on our backs, put our feet up and rest...

Boomerang Joy

VERSE FOR TODAY: **2 Corinthians 9:11**

You will be made rich in every way so that you can be generous on every occasion, and through us your generosity will result in thanksgiving to God.

MR. PHILLIP SIMMONS resides in Charleston, South Carolina. He is a master ironworker, a National Treasure of the Smithsonian Institute. Magazine articles have featured his work. His unique style makes his work highly sought after in all of Charleston, many parts of the South, and around the world. Despite his many accolades, he lives a simple life. Although retired, he still works from the original blacksmith shop behind his modest home. Not concerned about riches, Mr. Simmons is astounded over the fuss about him.

On a bus tour to his home and shop, tourists asked him about his giving to others, especially his nieces and nephews by supporting their college educations. His response as he stood on the tour bus full of tourists in awe of his accomplishments, was simple and insightful. He indicated it's a strange thing. He stated, he just keeps **giving and giving** and just keeps **getting and getting** more and more. Imagine— the more he gives the more he keeps getting—not only money and recognition but also **JOY**. The foundation established in his name will extend that **joy** for generations to come.

I call that boomerang joy. A boomerang, a simple, flat, curved implement, is amazing. Throw it, and it comes back to the thrower. Mr. Simmons' **joy** in giving becomes someone else's **joy**, which gives him more **joy** to give to others. This boomerang **joy** springs up when we honor God by giving and spreading **joy** to others. Spreading God's **joy** becomes our **joy**.

Spreading **joy** can become contagious. The multiplier effect comes into being when we help those who have not. Thanksgiving meals, Christmas toys, the **joy** of seeing the **joy** on someone else's face are primary motivators for helpers and caregivers who give freely of themselves. Giving grudgingly is not really giving and robs one of the boomerang joy-for the spirit in which you spread **joy** to others determines how **joy** comes back to you.

NUGGET FOR TODAY: Today I will toss the boomerang with joy!

PRAYER FOR TODAY: Loving God, the God of all Joy, may we find joy in giving to others with the simplicity and spirit of Mr. Simmons. May we experience the boomerang joy of knowing that the more we give, the more we receive. You created the physical laws of nature that make a simple implement, the boomerang, return to the thrower. Help us to find opportunities to share with no expectation of a return, but knowing that You engage in the boomerang effect, giving us blessings and joy too numerous to calculate. May the joy we spread burst forth in joy to others as it makes its way throughout the universe. May we be eternally blessed by what we give and what comes back to us…

What's A Ric Rac?

VERSE FOR TODAY: John 15:5

I am the vine, you are the branches. If a man remains in me and I in him, he will bear much fruit.

EVEN THOUGH MY Christmases while growing up in Georgia were simple, every one was special. The eldest of seven children, I remember Christmas Eve was a burst of excitement that we could hardly contain. We spent a restless night wondering what Santa would bring. We had no problem rising early on Christmas day, rushing to find our stockings stuffed with inexpensive toys that were the highlights of our day. One toy that we got year after year was what we called a ric rac. It was a paddle with a long rubber band, with a little red ball attached to it. The player would put the ball on the paddle, hit it and try to keep it going.

That ric rac provided endless hours of play and led to stiff competitions to see who could keep the ball going the longest. A player could be quickly eliminated though—if the rubber band broke and the ball went flying off in the distance or possibly in the woods near our house. We became creative repairers. If we could find the ball, we would tie a knot in the rubber and, we'd be back in the game, albeit with less bounce left. Sometimes we would find another rubber band that worked, but not as well as the original. A player could stay in the game as long as he or she could keep connected.

If we couldn't make a successful repair, being the resourceful children that we were, we would find other ways to use the remains. The paddle could be used in other ways, such as a makeshift badminton paddle. The ball could be used to play jacks; but there was little use for the rubber band if it became detached from the "vine". So the aim of the game was to stay connected. Keeping the rubber band, ball, and paddle intact led to much fruit, hours of playing, finding creative ways to bounce the ball-up, down, back, forth-bearing the fruit of endless hours of wild abandon as we played in the hot Georgia sun. If we remain connected to the Vine, we will bear much fruit.

NUGGET FOR TODAY: Today I will stay connected to the Vine.

PRAYER FOR TODAY: Dear God, You are our Vine. If we become disconnected, where will we get our nurturance and sustenance? Lord without You we would be truly lost. Help us to stay connected to You, the Source of our strength. Help us to gain strength from You. We know there will be seasons of pruning; we submit to your pruning. Prune us to make us stronger and better for Your work. Help us to bear fruit in all that we do; help us to abide in You, knowing our bounty will be plentiful if we stay connected...

Spring Fling!

VERSE FOR TODAY: Song of Songs 2:11-12

See! The winter is past; the rains are over and gone. Flowers appear on the earth; the season of singing has come ...

DURING THE COLD of winter when the snow covers the ground, the days seem to have more than their share of darkness. With the long days of little sunlight, a relatively newly defined phenomenon, *Seasonal Affective Disorder* (SAD), infuses our vocabulary. We are weighed down with layers of clothes. The birds are scarce, and the trees and shrubs appear as skeletons—it's hard to anticipate the coming of spring. But even though the cold of winter seems to freeze the life out of everything, the cycle of life is still happening beneath the cold earth.

The tulips and other bulbs that we plant during late fall need the cold of winter to burst forth in all their radiance in the spring. Even if we try to grow bulbs in containers (force them), they need to spend time in a cold refrigerator or garage, for example before they can bloom. Trees and shrubs need this time of winter rest to store up energy to sprout leaves, blossoms, and ultimately fruit.

But, inevitably, in its own time spring bursts forth with a *spring fling!* A time of dormancy is over. So, I encourage you to have a spring fling! As helpers, may we use the rhythm of the seasons to help those we serve and care for survive the cold, wintry times of their lives. May we prepare them to spring forth when the time comes to flower and to bear the fruit of meeting their goals, and progressing toward healing and wholeness.

Fling away the doldrums
Fling away the ho-hums
Fling away the despair
Spring is in the air!

Fling away the depression
Fling away the cold's obsession
Fling away winter's snare
Spring is in the air.

Fling away the sofa's grip
Fling away the nasal drip
Fling away the "I don't care"
Spring is in the air.

NUGGET FOR TODAY: Regardless of the season, I will have a spring fling!

PRAYER FOR TODAY: Dear God, the One who created the order of the earth, You knew the joy we would find after a season of winter's cold grip. You knew we would experience the doldrums and other maladies during the winter; but You reserved the beauty of spring and the songs of the birds to bring us spring joy. As soon as the first crocus springs forth, even though it may have one day of joy only to be covered with ice and snow, it still pops its head back up saying, "I survived the cold ground." So, Great Creator, help us to lead those we serve through the wintry pain to the spring beauty and joy of what they can be when they burst forth in due time…

Endless Love

VERSE FOR TODAY: Romans 8:38-39

For I am convinced that neither death nor life, neither angels nor demons, neither the present, nor the future, nor any powers, neither height nor depth, nor anything else in creation, will be able to separate us from the love of God that is in Christ Jesus our Lord.

WHEN I WAS a child, we used to sing a song about God-His being so high you can't get over Him, so low you can't go under Him, so wide you can't get around Him. That song seems to be a reflection of this verse.

What comfort! We can't be separated by :

DEATH	Nor	LIFE
ANGELS	Nor	DEMONS
PRESENT	Nor	FUTURE
ANY POWERS		
HEIGHT	Nor	DEPTH
ANYTHING ELSE IN ALL CREATION		

According to these words, try as hard as we may, we can't be separated from God's love. This passage runs the gamut of things that make God's love inescapable. The list presented here as well as any descriptors or extreme analogies we could come up with would not refute this inescapable Love. Believers can go to the highest heights or the lowest depths; still God's love would be there. Nothing that man could conceive or create could separate us from the ultimate manifestation of the Love of God. We can have complete confidence that for us it is impossible for human powers or anything else to separate us from God.

The kids say, "God loves you and there is nothing you can do about it." Even if we fail to love God, or fail to love ourselves, God's Love remains. There are no strings attached. John 15:10 tells us that Christ invites all to abide in his love. God is no respecter of persons.

We are invited to:

**BASK, RESIDE, SOAK UP, BE INFUSED WITH,
ENJOY, BE INVIGORATED BY... GOD'S LOVE.**

Perhaps love is the one complete element that permeates the helping process. Although helpers are cautioned regarding having feelings of love for their clients, love is possibly the force that drives helpers and caregivers to spend countless hours in service for others. In fact, helpers must "love" what they do. Long hours, low pay, few rewards, even repeat offenders are the payoffs for many. But the inescapable Love of God is often the fuel that keeps many helpers on the job despite the highs and lows, demons present and future, or anything else in creation that gets in the way. To experience this love is to experience joy. We should breathe deeply to take in the scents of the fragrance of love that is offered by the one who is Love: God.

NUGGET FOR TODAY: I will remember that God is Love and I will take advantage of that love.

PRAYER FOR TODAY: God, You are Love. You love us whether we want it or think we deserve it or not. You love us enough to let us make our mistakes and think we are making things happen. You love us enough to let us stray from Your presence. But You are always ready to pull us back to Your bosom that overflows with love. God, we thank You that there are no strings attached to Your love; everyone regardless of status or station is equally loved. We know we make You sad when we even fail to love ourselves, making it difficult for us to love others. Father, we pray that we can have a new-found appreciation of Your love and that we will shower that endless love on others...

Think Snow!

VERSE FOR TODAY: Job 38:22

Have you entered the storehouses of the snow…

AFTER PROMOTING SPRING Fling! earlier, it may seem a departure to suggest that we think snow! However, I have found snow to be a fascinating creation. Snow is formed when a particle of dust passes through the atmosphere and attaches to a droplet of water and freezes. No two snowflakes are the same. Most of the well-known Biblical references to snow are regarding its whiteness:

Psalm 51:7	*Wash me and I will be whiter than snow*
Isaiah 1:18	*Though your sins are like scarlet, they will be whiter than snow*
Daniel 7:9	*His clothing was white as snow*
Matthew 28:3	*His appearance was like lightning; and his clothes were white as snow*

Snow is the standard by which all whiteness is measured. But how does snow become so white? The intriguing descriptors "treasury or storehouses" of snow reveal the Lord's omnipotence—Only He has the recipe for its whiteness. During the harsh winters in Cleveland, Ohio when the snow seems endless, I often wonder how massive is this storehouse? But thank God that He doesn't dump all the snow on us at once. We would never survive this white, powdery onslaught that would bury us all. The capacity of all the snow making machines in all the ski lodges in the entire world would not compare with this treasury. This phrase "storehouses of snow" is a metaphor that refers to the things we humans can't fathom or have no control over. God uses the whiteness of snow to contrast with the scarlet of sin. God's grace and mercy are part of the cleaning supplies. Hyssop, which was used in ritual cleansing, is also included. Asking for cleansing is the first step to healing and wholeness.

As helpers in the Snow Belt areas especially, we know the power of snow. A few flakes-just flakes and flakes and flakes— become inches, even more flakes and flakes—become feet, more and more flakes and flakes—become a blizzard-enough to bring a city to a halt. Snowplows and salt crews work overnight and overtime, clearing the snow—sometimes to no avail; their paths are covered as soon as they make them. Cars can't drive, planes can't fly, and people can't walk.

But beholding the awesome beauty of a snow-covered forest or a snow-capped mountain, or looking out on a powdery wonderland can make up for the distress snow can cause. Contemplating each flake as it makes its journey to the earth can be a time of meditation and reflection and thanksgiving. So *think snow*!—the power of one, the determination of each single flake to find its rightful place, to make its single contribution in making a blizzard, and you will have to realize the treasury is controlled by the Divine Snow Maker.

NUGGET FOR TODAY: Today I will celebrate the determination of each snowflake to find its rightful place.

PRAYER FOR TODAY: Dear Heavenly Snowmaker, let us realize the power and determination of one flake. As a flake falls to the ground it adds a little by itself, but as it is joined by the other flakes from Your treasury, it has the power to bring a nation to a halt. We pray that we can learn to appreciate the uniqueness of each flake, reflecting on our own uniqueness. We can be thankful that You don't allow the whole treasury of snow to fall on us at once—You give us doses as You see fit. We thank You that You have given us some meager human means to deal with the snow: shovels, snow blowers, snow plows, and salt. Help us to use similar meager means to help those we serve shovel a path on the sidewalk, or plow through a blizzard, or to use salt to help them get traction and keep the road clear. Thank You for helping us realize that even snow doesn't last always…

A Drop in The Bucket

Verse for Today: Luke 15:4

Then Jesus told them this parable: "Suppose one of you has a hundred sheep and loses one of them. Does he not leave the ninety-nine in the open country and go after the lost sheep until he finds it?"

Drip...... drip...... drip
Drop...... drop...... drop
How much will it be
Before it stops?

Drip...... drip...... drip
Drop...... drop......drop
Each ONE drop
Can add up to lots.

Have you ever had a leak and used a bucket to catch the drip? Sure enough, if the drops continue, in no time, the bucket will overflow. This is a parable that stresses the importance of **ONE**. Found in the Gospel of Luke, we are told about a man who had 100 sheep and lost **ONE**. He left the other 99 sheep to search for the lost **ONE**. For him, his herd was not complete without the lost **ONE**. Likewise, a woman lost **ONE** of her silver coins. She searched, lit a lamp, and examined every corner until she found the **ONE** lost coin (Luke 15:8-10).

Both of these parables provide insight into the importance of **ONE**. Sometimes helpers have to prioritize or almost "triage" as they serve their clients. How does one deal with competing needs in case loads or patient loads? Can we follow the example in the parable whereby we put our time and energy into helping each **ONE**—at least for a spell—while the other **ONES** are temporarily put on hold? Sometimes—maybe, but certainly not always, as the phone rings, the referrals keep coming, the needs keep changing. How does a helper devote adequate attention to each **ONE?**

If we look at the steady drip, drip, drop, drop analogy, as small successes gradually mount; they will become a bucketful of successful outcomes. Just as the man rejoiced over the lost sheep-God rejoices and we should rejoice over the **one** who repents, the **one** who is helped, the **one** who moves toward healing. Just as the woman rejoiced over finding her lost coin, we can rejoice over the **one** who entered a treatment center, the mother who got her children back, **one** who received a diploma or certificate, **one** who was cured from cancer, **one** who joined the church, **one** who can say "I am a survivor." With each "drop in the bucket" —drops of small successes can give reason to celebrate the importance of **ONE** and focus on the **One** who bears our burdens…

Drip…….drip…….drip
Drop……….drop……….drop
Each one, when added to the other
Becomes more than a drip or a drop and……….
Before we know it, our bucket spills over the top.

NUGGET FOR TODAY: I will focus on the patter of drip, drop knowing before long the successes will overflow.

PRAYER FOR TODAY: Dear Heavenly Father, please help us to understand the power of one; help us to understand that every drop in the bucket, every small success, every accomplishment is a testament to Your goodness and grace. Help us to teach those we help to build on and celebrate each success with praise and thanksgiving. Help us to grasp onto each small success, those drops in the bucket. Help us to know when to focus on the **ONE**, leaving the others in Your care until we can return to them. Help us to rejoice when the bucket overflows and it's time to let go. When the time comes, give us wisdom to know to empty the bucket whether healing or transformation has occurred in our eyes or not. Help us to rejoice over the **ONE** as enthusiastically as we would for the 99 others…

Weed People

VERSE FOR TODAY: **Matthew 13:24-26, 29**

Jesus told them another parable: "The kingdom of heaven is like a man who sowed good seed in his field. But while everyone was sleeping his enemy came and sowed weeds among the wheat and went away."

When asked by his servants do you want us to pull up the weeds, he said no because while you are pulling up the weeds, you may also pull up the wheat (Verse. 29).

ANY GARDENER KNOWS the characteristics of weeds. One thing that always amazes me is the way weeds operate. They can grow in the most unlikely places—sidewalks or driveway cracks, along the roadside, in mountain crevices, along the seashore…they will find a way. All too often, they grow in the midst of our lawns, our corn fields and wheat fields, our gardens, flower boxes, our flower pots…

One source of consternation for a gardener is that s-o-o often weeds take on the characteristics of our precious flowers, vegetables, and other plants. How many times have we pulled up a "weed" only to realize it was a small seedling we planted? How often have we sprayed "weed killer" on what we later realized was a flower? How often do weeds sprout up among our tomato plants looking just like tomatoes; or how often do marigold look-alikes fool us? Many times the weeds are so entangled with the plants both are damaged and killed during our attempts to separate them. How often do the weeds choke out the good plants?

This parable has many implications for the helper. First, we are likely to find that just as we plant successes and positives within those we help, someone comes along and sows weeds among our successes—creating a need to re-seed. Secondly, how difficult is it to weed out those negative influences among those we help without somehow disturbing their fragile roots and anchors in the meantime? Thirdly, how often might we mistake the good among those we help as weeds, or fail to see the potential of a seedling that we pulled up? Weeding, thinning, pruning, and fertilizing are important tasks for the gardener. Sometimes, it's important to let the plant grow for a while to allow us to really determine if what appears to be a weed is really a weed or a beautiful flower.

NUGGET FOR TODAY: **Weeding is a necessary part of planting successes.**

PRAYER FOR TODAY: Dear Master Gardener, weeding is hard. How do we know when to weed and to feed? How do we know when to prune or when to let our precious plants freely grow? Lord, we ask that You help us to remove all those weeds that choke the life out of those we serve and care for. Help us to protect those precious fragile seedlings with love, water, a dose of fertilizer, and tender loving care. Help us to realize that thinning is sometimes necessary. Also, help us to know when to transplant. Give us the discernment to know when harvest time is appropriate. Help us plant seeds of hope ...

Clean The Closet

VERSE FOR TODAY: Psalm 55:22

Cast your cares on the LORD and he will sustain you; and he will never let the righteous fall.

OVER THE YEARS, closets have evolved from being nails or pegs on a wall, to a tiny cubbyhole, to elegant rooms with organized sections and seats. Now they have dressing areas and well-designed storage areas. Closets have tried to keep up with our insatiable demand for more stuff-clothes, shoes, outerwear, underwear, sportswear …

The number and sizes of closets are main features that add to the value of a property. Closets can sway a buyer from one property to another. Closets are for storing clothes, but metaphorically they can also be viewed as repositories where we pile up our burdens, where we hide our true selves, where we put away things we don't want to see, where we hide things we don't want others to see.

Closets can be the places where we stash our "junk" alongside the good stuff. Sometimes our closets house so much junk we can't even see the good stuff. We can't even see that perfect blouse to perk up an old suit, or that new pair of shoes that would add a special touch to an outfit, or that special accessory, scarf, or tie that can lift our spirits.

Why do we amass so much stuff? Simple: we tend to expect each item to make us look good, or feel important—make us happy. But all too often this stuff becomes just stuff—fueling our desire to accumulate more and increase our indebtedness in the process. As helpers, we may need to clean out the clutter, rearrange our space, and come to terms with our need to accumulate things.

When working with those we serve, we may need to help them clean their closets. We need to help rid them of burdens—the dreary and dull items that weigh them down; the old clothes they wear for comfort, rather than facing the challenges of change—the change that comes with a truly needed "new outfit." We may need to help rid them of the burdens of the "too small" outfits they are keeping just in case. Most of all, we may need to help them cast off all that lurks in the closet and hinders them from making positive steps, from keeping their eyes on the prize, and making it to the finish line. So rather than put on layer upon layer of heavy clothing, we need to help those we care for cast off these burdens. We need to realize that some closet-cleaning is needed.

NUGGET FOR TODAY: **It's time to clean the closet.**

PRAYER FOR TODAY: Dear Burden Bearer, You are the only one who can truly help us to clean our closets. You never treat us as cast offs, nor cast asides, but rather as Your special children who sometimes need to clean our closets. Lord, we collect so much, hold on to so much, and try to find happiness and meaning in so many things rather than You. We try to carry our own loads and bear our own burdens. We hide beneath layer upon layer of clothes. We are reluctant to shed them because we feel vulnerable without them—open to the prying eyes of others, causing us to retreat to our secret closets. Lord, help us to free ourselves of that which hinders us; help us to cast our burdens on You so that our closets can be special spaces—ones that store things to help us get dressed to face another day...

Car Wash Faith

VERSE FOR TODAY: James 1:6

But when he asks, he must believe and not doubt, because he who doubts is like a wave of the sea, blown and tossed by the wind.

WHEN I WAS growing up in Midland, a small town outside Columbus, Georgia, I never recall going to a car wash. We would pull our cars up to the faucet, hose the car down, soap it up good, rinse the soap off, and often let the southern sun dry it off. So, imagine after moving to Cleveland, Ohio, during those harsh winters when the snow and salt made it hard to even tell what color the car was, and the water would freeze as you sprayed it on, it was necessary to go to a car wash to remove the salt and road grime. Well, that was a new experience for me.

Even to this day, I realize I lack the skills to drive onto the conveyor without the help of the attendant. I wonder what they think of such "lady drivers?" But, once the attendant collects the money for the many options: chassis bath, wax, wheel brightener … there are instructions: windows up, car in neutral, foot off the brake—off I go.

Ride with me on this car wash journey. All sorts of thoughts go through my mind every time. Once the brushes start (touchless washes—using powerful water sprays are the latest) and the water pours on the car, I can't see a thing. Tons of "what ifs" crop up: "What if I run into the car in front of me; what if I can't stop when it's done, what if I left a window cracked, what if water gets on the engine, what if the car behind me can't stop?"

During my first solo car wash, I wanted to put my foot on the brake, but I just went with the flow. I had to have *car wash faith*. I had to trust the attendant to guide me onto the conveyor; I had to trust the conveyor to move me along at the right pace; I had to trust the mechanisms to wash my car, even the chassis, and to dry the car when finished.

So often we need to teach those we help to have car wash faith—to put the car in neutral and let it roll. They need the faith to drive without any doubt and to have steadfastness and not be tossed about by the brushes and torrents of warm sudsy, high-powered water that's needed to get our cars clean and spotless—at least until the next snowstorm. Even the old, beat-up cars look much better after the car wash. A car wash can give the feeling of being tossed about, feelings of uncertainty, but faith in the One who can calm the sea is a great assurance that we can come out looking like new.

Nugget for Today: I will put it in neutral and go with the flow.

Prayer for Today: Dear Calmer of the Sea and Anchor for those tossed and driven by the wind and rains, we pray for car wash faith. We trust the skills of the attendant who takes our money, guides us onto the conveyor. We trust the water, brushes, and soap to clean off the salt, dirt, grime, and hassles from the roads of life. Likewise, we trust You as we go through the car washes of life. We pray for faith to put the car in neutral, take our foot off the brake. We expect to emerge clean, shiny and dry as we go on our way. May we emerge as shining vessels, gleaming in Your glory and exhibiting a new sense of newness, confidence, and faith...

Polluted Water

Verse for Today: James 3:11

Can both fresh water and salt water flow from the same spring?

This verse is part of James' exhortations regarding the tongue. The tongue is described as a small organ, "a little member", or "small part of the body" (James 3:5) but capable of producing much hurt, harm, chaos, and confusion. The tongue can lead to fights, wars and brokenness. It can also lead to defilement. In fact, some experts say that verbal abuse is the most insidious form of abuse, because words of the tongue can break one's spirit and lower one's self-esteem, can eliminate the desire to break free; thus it can hold one mentally and consequently physically hostage.

Just as a small amount of yeast can cause a loaf of bread to rise, a small amount of tainted or polluted water with its microscopic bacteria and microorganisms renders a spring unclean. It can take the freshness away, leading to stagnation. A bad drop of water, like a negative comment can pollute one's desires.

As helpers, we must ask ourselves two main questions: Are we sending double messages? Are we lauding praise on those we serve one day or session, and making non-supportive admonishments the next? Secondly, we must question our attitudes. Do we speak with forked tongues—saying one thing when we mean another? Or, are we filled with hypocrisy, not practicing what we preach?

Clients can sense if we are caring and sincere. Earlier, James gives some instructions that can benefit the helper. In James 1:19 he states: "Be swift to hear [or listen] and slow to speak." Sometimes it is hard for those we help to clearly articulate their feelings and situations. Having a listening ear for what is said and unsaid is important.

When clients do share, let us respond with kind words and understanding. Let our sentiments be like fresh water springing up from the core of our being. Let the polluted water that may lurk beneath the surface be so diluted with freshness that pollution ceases to exist. Words can harm; words can heal. Let us relate to one another and our clients from springs that have been cleansed with water from the eternal springs that run deep, rooted and overflowing with God's love.

Nugget for Today: I will not let polluted water taint my spring of freshness.

Prayer for Today: Dear Creator of Fresh Springs of Water, may we live in constant awareness of the impact of one drop of polluted water. May our fresh water always gush forth so strongly that it dilutes and eliminates any tainted water that lurks beneath the surface. May we sincerely speak words of understanding and support and turn off the spigot of any undesirable thoughts and negative words that may be waiting to spring forth. May we not speak polluted words of confusion and contradiction. Rather, may we dam up those springs of freshness so that we can offer a fresh drink to anyone who is thirsty for support and healing...

Get New Luggage

VERSE FOR TODAY: Job 11:18

You will be secure, because there is hope; you will look about you and take your rest in safety.

AFTER SEPTEMBER 11, 2001 also known as 9/11, airports in the United States and consequently around the world imposed new policies and procedures—new regulations for travelers. In addition to the new requirements for passengers themselves, stricter search procedures were implemented for baggage. It was all about safety. For me specifically, these changes required that I think carefully about what I packed. Magazine articles, and television shows presented several suggestions such as putting underwear and other personal items in plastic bags to avoid their being touched by TSA (Transportation Security Administration) staff. To avoid delays, they suggested putting shoes on the top and reminded travelers to anticipate the possibility that their luggage could be physically searched.

The latter suggestion really caused me to rethink what I would pack. So, often my luggage—although neatly packed—would be stuffed to the brim. After a hasty unpacking by agents, I thought I may never be able to re-pack in a hurry. So the law of parsimony became my new standard. Besides standard cosmetics and items that I always carried and needed, I began to weigh the merits of each piece that I packed. I found a system that revolved around a few standard pieces with each item meeting three criteria to make the cut: lightweight and pack-able, not bulky, and coordinating with at least two other items.

In fact, because of my new strategy, I decided to buy new luggage. The big Pullman that I struggled with was replaced by a smaller, lighter, easier to manage one. I found creative ways to coordinate my outfits. I found I needed fewer shoes and could even have room to bring a new coordinating piece or two home with me. Yes, according to Homeland Security and the Transportation Security Administration, new rules and regulations were needed for safety-new guidelines for luggage and new rules for travelers. However, safety and security are best assured when we trust the One who has all of eternity in His hands. Get new luggage, unload the unnecessary, repack, taking only what you need for the journey. Trust in the God of transportation safety and security to ensure your safe travels.

NUGGET FOR TODAY: **I will take only what I need.**

PRAYER FOR TODAY: Dear Lord, the only One who can assure our safety and security, we will pack with You in mind. You give us assurances that You will always take care of us and make us to dwell in safety. You control the flights, the schedules, and all of our comings and goings. As we think about what we should pack, may we choose things that do not weigh us down, things that help us to easily navigate the airports and terminals, the baggage claim and the ground transportation of our daily lives. Most of all help us to rest in the knowledge that You will see us safely to our destination. Let us get new luggage, and fill it to overflowing with those things that have eternal security...

Lighten the Load

VERSE FOR TODAY: Matthew 11:28-30

Come to me, all you who are weary and burdened, and I will give you rest. Take my yoke upon you and learn from me, for I am gentle and humble in heart, and you will find rest for your souls. For my yoke is easy and my burden is light.

Action Verbs: **COME, TAKE, LEARN, FIND.**

THE ACTION VERBS and descriptors in this text provide a good formula for lightening the load. In this text, Jesus was referring to the burdens imposed by those trying to follow the religious responsibilities to the letter of the law. Often in the lives of helpers, the burdens, or the letter of the law come in the form of personnel practices and work rules, restrictive policies, unmanageable caseloads, competing demands: meetings versus counseling session, versus paperwork, the list goes on. Many days go by in a blur and the stress of the labor (daily struggles) and the burdens (overworked, overloaded, never enough time, never enough resources) are taxing and all consuming.

The reference to a yoke seems all too fitting. Oftentimes days are spent like farm animals that are harnessed together, endlessly plowing the fields, being even too tired to rest at the end of the day. But the action verbs in this passage make all the difference.

COME:

Come, cast your cares on Me
Come, count on My energy
Come, be replenished
Come, find the resources you need.
LEARN FROM ME

TAKE

Take off the yoke
Take off the stress
Take from the storehouse of blessings
LEARN FROM ME

FIND

Find the rest you need
Find the strength you need
Find more hours in the day
Find your strength in Me.
LEARN FROM ME

Everyday, *come* to the "Burden Bearer", everyday, *take* off a little, and before you know it, you will *find*—the load will be lighter, the load will be more bearable, the load will be more manageable, the journey will be more bearable, and yes, probably without noticing it, your yoke will be easier and the burden lighter. Helpers, let's also use this formula to help ourselves and find rest for our souls. **Learn from the Burden Bearer.**

NUGGET FOR TODAY: **Today I will come, take, find.**

PRAYER FOR TODAY: Lord, You are the Burden Bearer. How can we make it without You? How can we even manage the demands of life unless we **come, take, and find**? What a consolation it is to know we no longer have to bear our own burdens. Thank You for these comforting words and the visual image of a yoke—realizing that You can bear our burdens much better than we. Lord, we will lighten the load. We hope to **come** to You to meet our needs, to let you **take** off our burdens and struggles, so that we can **find** rest in the assurance that You are a gentle Savior who provides what we need along this journey of being a helper and caregiver…

Godly DNA

Verse for Today: Exodus 34:6

And he passed in front of Moses, proclaiming, "the LORD, the LORD the compassionate and gracious God, slow to anger, abounding in love and faithfulness...

Over the past few years, there has been an explosion of the use of DNA. In fact, this acronym is so common, I suspect few even know that the letters stand for *deoxyribo nucleic acid*. DNA has been used to nail suspects and to reverse convictions, to identify bodies, and to determine family lineage, to name a few ways this technology has become a regular part of our society.

In I Kings 3:16-26, we see how Solomon's wisdom helped him settle a dispute in the story of two mothers who each had a baby son. When the one son was smothered by his mother, the mother tried to claim the other child as hers. Solomon used his God-given wisdom and suggested cutting the living child in two, giving a half to each mother. The real mother cried for Solomon to give the child to the other woman, thus revealing the true mother. Today, DNA would probably be used to solve such a dispute and determine the real mother. Just a small sample of one's unique identifier—DNA can be used to determine identity, to connect one to a crime, or to solve a mystery.

But, how does one use DNA to determine a Godly person? If one were on trial, what about **Exhibit A** would lead to Godly DNA? The Lord described His unique characteristics as He passed in front of Moses in a cloud. Compassionate, gracious, slow to anger, abounding in love and faithfulness. Do we exhibit these characteristics as we help others? We should, for we are children of God; we should bear His DNA as a testament to the unique qualities that define a helper.

Nugget for Today: Today I will exhibit Godly DNA.

Prayer for Today: Dear God, what an awesome, humbling, and sometimes scary thought—we bear Your DNA. We use the acronym loosely, but looking at our heritage, we can trace our lineage to You the Great and Awesome God. As the bearers of Your DNA, may we strive every day to embody You. May our words, action, deeds, and thoughts display love, compassion, graciousness, kind words. May we turn from anger and wrath and exhibit peace and calm in every situation. May we demonstrate love and faithfulness, may we be proud to present **Exhibit A**, Godly DNA…

Divine Job Description

VERSE FOR TODAY: Colossians 3:12

Therefore, as God's chosen people, holy and dearly loved, clothe yourselves with compassion, kindness, humility, gentleness, and patience.

OVER THE YEARS, the process of finding a job has vastly changed. Although the newspapers still have a help wanted section, and people still post help wanted signs, many of today's jobseekers use the World Wide Web to search for jobs and post their résumés. They may even participate in phone, online, or remote interviews. Employers post their job openings on websites and electronic job boards. Search engines guide the job seeker through thousands of possibilities. The job seeker can connect to openings worldwide.

In searching for openings, what might helpers look for in want ads or job descriptions? In addition to wanting to know the job title, the company address, and the salary, job seekers want to read a job description. This is used to find the match between person and position.

But helpers need to have some unique words or phrases in their job descriptions. The characteristics are based on the characteristics of God, who epitomizes what a helper should be as stated in the verse for today. How can helpers exhibit these attributes in their daily work? Can we be described as exhibiting ***compassion, kindness, humility, gentleness, and patience?***

We may not feel that it's appropriate to list these traits on our résumés, but we should strive to live them out as we go about the task of helping others, thereby filling out the requirements presented in God's want ad. As we dress for work every day, in addition to our garments, we should clothe ourselves in the spiritual characteristics that exhibit God's characteristics. As others physically see and interact with us, as we are the hands and feet of Jesus, let God's job description be permanently posted on our human resources bulletin boards and on our websites, so jobseekers worldwide would want to apply for a helping position.

Nugget for Today: I will exhibit the characteristics of God's help wanted posting.

Prayer for Today: Loving God, help us to develop divine job descriptions. We pray that Your glory and Your characteristics will show through us and in all that we do. Let us embrace the characteristics that make us fit to apply for the position of helper as described in Your want ad: *compassion, kindness, humility, gentleness, and patience*. When we check the bulletin board for that perfect job and when we complete an application, help us to be comfortable enough in an interview to describe those characteristics that represent You. Let us be eager to do "other duties as assigned," and may we be the perfect applicant for the awesome job of *helper...*

Water Minded

Verse for Today: Psalm 42: 1-2

As the deer pants for streams of water, so my soul pants for you O God. My soul thirsts for God, the living God …

Water is all the rage these days. Growing up in Georgia, early on our water was supplied by a well. We didn't have city-supplied tap water. Instead, we enjoyed the refreshing coolness of well water on a hot summer day. This water also made yummy lemonade and refreshing iced tea. Now bottled water has become the rage. We were familiar with Perrier-and perhaps a few other brands; then came a deluge of bottled water, some from springs, some purified. One has to really read the labels to reveal the variety of water sources.

Anyway, it has become "chic" to have a bottle of water all the time. Now, water is a billion-dollar industry. Some don't travel without it. Imagine their dismay during an elevated terror alert in August 2006 after a suspected terror plot. Travelers had to discard all liquids—coffee and other beverages, medications, toiletries, and yes water.

Water comes flavored, enhanced with minerals, with enticing labels and catchy sayings. Still many don't drink enough. Water is the ultimate thirst quencher for the panting soul. To "pant" refers to a spiritual thirst for God. The deer pants for water, the helper and caregiver often pant for God. As a deer pants with an intense thirst for water from a cool stream, humans pant for living fountains of water, wells that never run dry. They pant for peace, for rest, for babbling brooks and thundering waterfalls, for cooling streams in the desert, for mist and morning dew, and rain drops for their parched souls.

Humans long for Jordan River and Red Sea and Galilee experiences. We long to linger in the Garden and rest by the River Euphrates. Yes, more than we realize it, we are water minded.

Water is valuable and sacred. Civilizations would vanish without access to water. Many take water for granted, but lately in many parts of the United States, communities are dealing with water shortages due to drought conditions. Even today, I read about a community that was restricting water usage to three hours per day. Water is a necessity, and just as the Woman of Samaria found her Living Water (John 4:10), we pant for the opportunity to drink from a fountain that never runs dry. Our physical, tired bodies pant for a warm bath or hot shower at the end of a dry, dusty day of helping others. We pant for the Living God.

NUGGET FOR TODAY: Today I will pant for the Living God.

PRAYER FOR TODAY: Lord, only You can quench the thirst in our souls. No cool spring water, well water, bottled water, distilled water, or tap water can satisfy our longing for You. Only You can quench our longing for peace, rest, and still waters. You made the small streams and You made the mighty oceans and seas. We long for You as we linger in the garden, as we need to be refreshed and renewed. Lord, we pray that those we help will know that tap water, bottled water or water drawn from a well quenches our human thirst, but that You alone, O God, are the answer when we have a spiritual thirst, when we "pant" for you. Thank You that Your well never runs dry, that it runs deep with "living water." May we have the courage to take a sip, and a sip, and a sip and drink up until You quench our panting and longings...

Spiritual Exercise

VERSE FOR TODAY: Acts 17:28

For in him we live, and move and have our being.

IT'S ALL THE rage—work that body!

Getting up, moving, and exercising, can be a challenge for some and perhaps an obsession for others. Pick up a catalog from a recreation center and the browser sees all kinds of exercises and fitness activities: *body sculpting, circuit training, Jazzercise, aerobocise, acquasise, cardio kick, Tai Chi, yoga.* There is a range of exercise dance types: the ever-popular *line dancing,* as well as *belly dancing, Latin dancing, even wedding party dance lessons.* And in addition to the standard weight training equipment, *treadmills, and stationary bikes*, options also include *bands, tubes, balls, and weight bars.* The workout terminology also includes activities such as *lunge, stretch, squat, lift, grape vine, curls.* Participants, ranging from *beginning to advanced,* are told to *inhale and exhale* in order to impact their *abs, gluts, biceps, and triceps.*

Work that body! Spiritual exercise seems so much simpler, just move, breathe, and have our being in Him. Helpers should be encouraged to develop a workout routine that includes a series of moves and repetitions that engage us with Him who gives to all, life and breath—every nation of man (Acts 17:26). No need to pull out the leotards and cross-trainer shoes; you don't have to buy any equipment, or videos. No need to worry about strains, tears, pulls. No need to build recreation centers, or tracks, or trails. Just exercise, move in Him. Take advantage of the opportunity to live and breathe in the One who gives life and breath to all. Yes, physical exercise is important, and we should maintain a daily physical routine, but spiritual exercise brings lasting results. Let's move and have our being in Him.

Nugget for Today: Today I will engage in *spiritual exercise.*

Prayer for Today: Dear Lord, the One in whom we live and move, and have our being, sometimes it seems that we are on the treadmill of life. We move faster; we adjust the incline; we add more time to the workout; we buy special equipment; but we often don't see any results. We tried the latest craze, even balancing on a big ball. We signed up for that popular exercise class. We even bought a series of tapes; we donned our fancy workout togs; but we still have not met our goals. So Lord, today we will engage in spiritual exercise. We will warm up by basking in Your love; our routine will include prayer, praise, worship, and thanksgiving—rejoicing that our being is in You. Then we will cool down by reaching out to You, for You are not far away. You give us the awesome assurance that we are Your offspring and our workout will be worth it...

Come Monday

VERSE FOR TODAY: Proverbs 27:1

Do not boast about tomorrow, for you do not know what a day may bring forth.

WHEN OUR MOTHER passed away several years ago, my siblings and I sat around reminiscing about her life, her witness, her words of wisdom, and the many things she taught us. We collected many of her favorite sayings such as "the early bird gets the worm," "haste makes waste," and one of special note: "don't put off for tomorrow what you can do today." She reminded us to always seize the moment, plan, prepare, and avoid procrastination.

During the past New Year, my siblings and I shared our New Year's Resolutions. We talked and laughed, and challenged each other to keep our individual resolutions. We also encouraged each other to keep his/her resolutions and promised to do reality checks during the year.

This year I was reminded of how often I've said; "Come Monday, I will… start exercising; I will start being more careful about what I eat; I will start saving more; I will start…this; stop that. I'm sure you have your own list of **starts and stops**.

Interestingly enough, it seemed to be Tuesday or Wednesday when I'd say come Monday—giving me a few more days before actually having to begin or follow through on my start or stop promise or resolution. After many come Mondays, I am still recommitting to some start or stop promises, but I have become more diligent about many.

As helpers, we may have many come Mondays. Mondays when we promised to start working on a certificate, license, or advanced degree. Or we may have made a resolution to get to work on time, or to start taking a lunch hour, or to take a vacation, or to stop taking work home, or to stop taking on clients' burdens, or to start being more vocal on clients' behalf. Helping others isn't easy, but hopefully you are reading this on a Saturday or Sunday, so that come Monday you can gradually develop a list of things to **start and to stop** that will help you become a better person inwardly (for yourself), and outwardly as you face the many challenges of helping others.

NUGGET FOR TODAY: **I will not put off for tomorrow what I can do today.**

PRAYER FOR TODAY: Dear Creator God, the One who holds all time in Your hands, the only One who knows what tomorrow holds, the only One who can orchestrate time, the only One who can help us make the most of each day, and the only One who can help us keep our promises, we pray that You will help us keep focused and adhere to our start and stop endeavors. We pray that You will help us face the challenges of each new tomorrow. We can't even say if we will live to see tomorrow, so we rely on Your strength to avoid putting off for tomorrow what we can indeed do today. We pray that come Monday, we will have already started on the road to doing what needs to be done. We want to **stop** those things that hold us captive and prevent us from making the most of each day. We want to **start** those things that make us a more productive, more efficient, and more effective helper. With Your help, come Monday, we will be able to …

Hide and Seek

VERSE FOR TODAY: Isaiah 55:6

Seek the LORD while he may be found; call on Him while he is near.

A FAVORITE GAME my family played while growing up in Georgia was "hide and seek." We grew up in a rural area with plenty of places to hide—in and around the house, the yard, the grounds, and the woods. It was easy to find a place to hide; and sometimes if you knew the habits of the "hiders," and looked for tell-tell signs, like leaves moving on a tree, or listened for giggles, it was easy for the "seekers" to find the "hiders."

Sometimes, if you were quiet and still, the seeker would be right by you, yet passed you by to seek for another hider. Sometimes I would get terrified thinking, "what if I hid myself too well; what if no one found me?" Silly me! Of course the object of the game was to not get found.

God makes it clear that He wants to be found. In fact this passage is two-fold. It tells us to seek the Lord; he's trying to be found. He's not playing childish games. He's not interested in hiding from us; he's interested in seekers.

Secondly, God lets us know He is never far away. He tells us to call on Him—He's near. He doesn't need to communicate by our modern-day methods—cell phones, e-mails, World Wide Web, no fancy personal data assistants, no gadgets hanging from our belts or purses—the only technology needed to make a connection is a willingness to seek Him.

So often those we serve will struggle with hiding and seeking; hiding their fears and weaknesses, and indiscretions; hiding that they "backslid" or "fell off the wagon," or they went back to an unhealthy situation. They may be seeking that one elusive treatment component or therapy, or word of wisdom, or positive affirmation that can help them to stick to their goals once and for all. I believe the action words of this passage can give clients stability in trying situations—seek the Lord and call on Him in any situation; they will find He is always near.

Nugget for Today: I will seek the Lord and call on Him today.

Prayer for Today: Dear God, the One who is never far away, thank You that You are <u>not</u> trying to hide from us. You can be in all places at all times, accessible to all human beings simultaneously and able to meet all of our needs with one wave of Your mighty hand, if we would only seek Your face. You don't play games of hide and seek. You are not trying to distance Yourself from us. We often hide from You and this hurts You because the invitation is always open. It hurts You to know that we seek any and everything before we seek and call on You. Help us to begin each day fully intent to seek You and to call on You along the way, and in our hour of need. Help us to stop playing childish games and take You at Your Word…

Rummage Sale

VERSE FOR TODAY: Romans 9:27

Though the number of the Israelites be like the sand by the sea, only the remnant will be saved.

EVERY THURSDAY IN the Inside & Out section of the *Cleveland Plain Dealer*, there is a list of upcoming rummage sales, flea markets, garage sales, and yard sales. People are constantly clearing out the clutter and trying to sell their un-useables or un-needed things—often for a fraction of the original cost. Everything must go! For most sellers, the joy and thrill that someone will buy their stuff is their motivation. For the buyers, the joy and thrill of getting a bargain is their attraction.

There are a couple of shows on television where people clean out their houses, put items on sale at an auction or yard sale to raise money to finance their reorganizing or remodeling projects. Watching antique shows and road shows can be quite intriguing. People bring in all sorts of things, sometimes having no idea they may have been holding on to a treasure. Some people have been pleasantly surprised or even shocked to find something they found in the attic or in someone else's trash was worth a great deal of money.

Not being a savvy collector, the question that keeps resonating through my mind is—how does one know what an item is worth? Not knowing the value makes one want to hold on to things just in case. Knowing what's trash and what's treasure is an art that may require years of tracking the history and value of an article. What is worth saving?

Sometimes the helper may be faced with what or who is worth saving. Is a client, a patient, a parishioner a lost cause because it seems he or she will never change, be cured, healed, or saved? We can take our attic finds to an appraiser to get an estimated value of an item. But, with human beings, we have to conclude that everyone is valuable, a treasure and worthy of being painted or polished, or buffed, re-framed, re-touched, and given a chance to shine. Everyone deserves the opportunity to reflect his or her true worth. In today's verse, only a remnant was saved, those who believed in God. However, since many we help are like the remnant, let's treat everyone as the treasure worth saving, ones whom God sees as valuable.

NUGGET FOR TODAY: I will consider everyone a treasure.

PRAYER FOR TODAY: Dear God, Only You can put a value on Your creations. Too often we casually look at people and try to determine their worth. We designate ourselves as earthly appraisers. Let us look upon everyone as a person of value—because You didn't make any junk. You didn't intend for anyone to be a cast off. Let us not be so quick to put our fellow humans on the curb for next day's rubbish pickup. Let us be ever mindful that those we consider trash, You treasure. Help us to pick up the cracked, the broken, the faded, and with Your love, give them new life. Help us to be rescuers and recyclers of those that society so casually casts aside…

Winning Team

VERSE FOR TODAY: Romans 8:31

What then shall we say in response to this? If God is for us, who can be against us?

IT IS MID-SPRING. We are in the midst of the National Basketball Association (NBA) playoffs. Little league teams are stepping up to the plate. America's favorite pastime—baseball will soon be in full swing.

Every team or individual athlete wants to feel the thrill of winning. For sure, some just play for the *fun of it*, and some just take *all of the fun out of it*. Over 30 years ago, when our son played Little League baseball—the pressure was always on. Whenever someone stepped to the plate, sometimes the stress was obvious and the agony of pressure from parents weighed the youngster down heavily. Everyone chanted, "Hey batter, batter, batter."

There was often a show on the sidelines as parents came close to engaging in fistfights. Unfortunately, there have been some serious altercations involving parents, some even ending in death. Teams, coaches, parents, players, and fans pray for their teams to win—and even pray that their wagers will make them winners.

No matter how the drafts, trades, talent scouts, agents, and team managers put their teams together, there is only one sure tried and true winning team—God's team. No matter how much we cheer, boo, hiss, chant, throw things on the field, or sing our rallying songs, God has already determined the final score. Our adversaries are powerless, so we should always exemplify that winning spirit.

With many of those we help, the game seems over before they get their turns at bat. An earthly referee has already called them out.

Strike three!   You're out of bounds!   Foul!

They hardly get any free throws, but are constantly being fouled. Or, they have fouled out before the toss of the ball. They can see the goal line, from a distance, but the ball is hardly ever passed to them.

Let's instill in those we help that it's not over till it's over. Many a game is won with the last shot or "hail Mary" pass. How often have we left the game early to beat the traffic only to find that the game took a turn and the final outcome changed after we left? On God's team, everyone has a turn at bat with the Heavenly Referee calling the strikes and balls. Everyone is given some balls, some free throws, and some free downs as they advance toward the goal line. The Head Coach makes sure everyone gets to play on the sure winning team—God's team.

Nugget for Today: Today I will suit up for God's team.

Prayer for Today: Dear Captain of the Winning Team, we want to sign up now! We also have some that we care for who want to be on Your team. We know that with You, three strikes are never out, because we can start over again and again. We know that we can't foul out or be benched if we're on Your team. Even though no one drafts us, we know that we are already chosen. Our Captain, we know that we, and those we care about, may be down at half time, but the second half is a new game. Let us not be as concerned about the half-time show as we are about our talks in the locker room with You, the Head Coach, calling the plays. Give us the strength, courage, wisdom, and stamina to take the baton, run the race, and cross the finish line—knowing that if You are for us, who cares who is against us. We're always on the winning team with You...

Survey your Surroundings

Verse for Today: Hebrews 12:1

Therefore, since we are surrounded by such a great cloud of witnesses, let us throw off every thing that hinders and the sin that so easily entangles, and let us run with perseverance the race is marked out for us.

This well-known scripture echoes with me of another of my mother's sayings. She continuously reminded us to be aware of those we associated with. She was not shy about telling us of the importance of the "company we keep."

In describing this section of Hebrews, we see the words: "the race of faith." In Chapter 11 of Hebrews, the "Honor Roll of Faith" is the subtitle. So faith permeates Chapters 11 and 12 of Hebrews. But, what about being surrounded by a cloud of witnesses? The book of Hebrews presents a long list of witnesses that span biblical history. Familiar names and their famous acts begin with Abel's offering to God, moves to Enoch, Noah, Abraham, Sarah, the Patriarchs—Isaac, Jacob, Joseph, then includes many others such as David and Rahab, the prostitute.

If I were to ask you to conduct a survey of your associations, who would be included in your cloud of witnesses? Who were your associates, influencers, mentors, role models—those who inspired you to become who you are? How would you describe the "company you keep?" Who were your detractors, or distracters like Sanballat and Tobiah who tried to get Nehemiah off course by constantly ridiculing him (Nehemiah 4:1-6)? Strengthened by Geshem, these two tried to lure Nehemiah away from God's work—aiming to distract him from his task (Nehemiah 6:1-4). Sanballat even spread slanderous reports that Nehemiah planned to become king.

On our life journey, we will meet all kinds of people. Some will want to permanently be included in our network—but when you survey your cloud of witnesses, who can stand the test of providing true support, well-meaning attitudes, and true friendship? Our surroundings can become clouded by those who disguise themselves as friends, but are intent on luring us away from our goals and our focus.

I have often been amazed by those who would deliberately try to keep clients from meeting their goals. They would set up roadblocks, use negative talk, and keep the client off-centered by backbiting, belittling, and begrudging their attempts to move forward. My dissertation was about social support networks. Findings supported the importance for persons to surround themselves with persons who could provide instrumental support (money, tangible resources), and affective support (positive words, kind acts). One's cloud of witnesses, and one's surroundings should help one successfully run the race that is uniquely his or hers.

NUGGET FOR TODAY: I will survey my surroundings and think about the company I keep.

PRAYER FOR TODAY: Loving God, Your Word provides a great list of witnesses—those who though imperfect, made the honor roll of faith. They ran their race with perseverance; they laid aside weights that would encumber them; and they ran their race with faith—focused on You. Let us have the stamina and determination of Nehemiah. May we not get side tracked, lured away from our task. Help us to survey the path that lies before us. May we clear our surroundings of anything, or anyone that hinders us, causes us to stumble, or weighs us down. May we be aware of the company we keep. May we remove the detractors from our list of associates and surround ourselves with a cloud of witnesses and examples that support and inspire us. May we help those we serve, develop a network of persons who strengthen, undergird and, lift them up...

GodSpace

VERSE FOR TODAY: Psalm 31:20

In the shelter of your presence you hide them.

IN THE *NELSON'S King James Reference Bible* I often use, commentary on this verse focuses on intimacy and friendship. Two words that spring forth from this Psalm describe God as a *fortress* and a *refuge*. These two words may conjure up opposing visions. A fortress is well planned, guarded, impenetrable (a shelter), and a refuge (God's presence) is a less-structured, safe, secure place to run to. Although this Psalm would be classified as one of lament, throughout, it also conveys trust and a hiding place.

Intimacy and friendship with God are also themes in this Psalm; thus, I am encouraging helpers to find a **GodSpace** if you don't have one. This space need not be created to be a fortress, nor does it have to be a nicely decorated, walled-off room. Rather, it should be a place where you can go to meditate, pray, study God's Word, sing soul stirring songs. It should foster quiet worship, should be a place that evokes the presence of God. In the case of the helper, it should be a space where the professional and the personal intersect. It should be the place where you hone your intuitive skills, where theories, and hypotheses, practice wisdom, and treatment methods are informed by the very presence and leading of God.

Several things should be placed in your **GodSpace**. A journal, perhaps a cross, a Bible, a rock to remind you of the steadfastness of God, pictures and collectibles —prayers, books, inspirational sayings, a flower, a candle, potpourri, whatever stirs your heart and causes you to reflect on the past, connect to the present, and anticipate the future should adorn your **GodSpace**. If your space is near a window, watch the birds; listen to their unique serenades. Watch other animals go about the business they were created to do. Watch the flowers progress from buds, to flowers, to seeds ready for another season of life. Watch the seasons change and the sun rise or set; reflect on the phases of the moon. Keep the door of your space (your heart) open for God to come in.

Nugget for Today: I will create and maintain my special GodSpace.

Prayer for Today: Dear God, we want to connect to You in so many ways. Often the days go by in a blur—**dayandeveningandnight** blending together. We often start out wanting to spend time with You but end up retiring from a busy day having had only casual thoughts of You, if any. We know we would be better helpers if we took time to meditate, spend time with You, discern what You would have us do, and how You would have us help each person we're responsible for. But, in our minds, we're often too busy. We want to create a **GodSpace**—a place for You to reside in our heart and a physical space with an open door to Your Presence. On some days, we may feel we need a well-protected fortress, while on others a refuge where we can hide in the secret place with You would do us well. We need intimacy and friendship with You to be at our best and to better serve those You put on our agenda. We will create a **GodSpace.** Beginning now You have an open invitation, You don't have to knock. Come in!…

New Wineskins

Verse for Today: Matthew 9:16-17

No one sews a patch of unshrunk cloth on an old garment, for the patch will pull away from the garment making the tear worse. Neither do men pour new wine into old wineskins. If they do, the skins will burst, the wine will run out and the wineskins will be ruined. No, they pour new wine into new wineskins, and both are preserved.

Trying to mix the old with the new doesn't always work. Oftentimes it may be best to begin anew. I recently purchased a new computer-USB (universal serial bus) port ready. Everything was connected; documents from the old computer were transferred; virus protection software was installed; the monitor and printer were connected; and I was set to go. I pulled up the most recent document I had worked on, clicked on the print icon and nothing happened. I tried again and again, but no go. The printer was serial port // or parallel, not USB. So my son found an adapter, connected the printer again, clicked on print and it worked. Well, my son knew some ways to tinker with the connections, something I would have to do every time. After a while, struggling to remember his instructions, I just decided it was time to buy a new printer.

I was trying to put new wine (computer) into old wineskins (printer). Just as I imagine it would be hard to retrofit a new automatic transmission to a car that was designed for a manual transmission, just as putting an addition onto a new house using old materials, even just as trying to make a ball point pen into an ink pen would hardly work, often it is best to start over—best to put new wine into new wineskins.

What are some messages found in this verse? Sometimes mixing the old with the new just won't work, if so, only for so long. Sometimes healing takes place best when old acquaintances, negative self-concepts, and limited vision are replaced with new realities, new, positive, refreshing people, images, and support. Persons bent on holding to the old ways, old habits, old patterns will not seek healing and restoration—they may be too comfortable with the old. The new brings challenges, changes, new worldviews. Let us help those we serve see new visions as they move toward healing and restoration. New energy and new visions together are less likely to tear away as would a new makeshift patch sewn onto old material.

NUGGET FOR TODAY: **Today I will focus on the new.**

PRAYER FOR TODAY: Dear Lord of the Vine, You created wine from the fruits of Your vineyards. You also gave us the wisdom to create vessels and containers such as wineskins. You gave us the wisdom to harvest the grapes; You formed the processes that allow fermentation to occur; and You created the drink that symbolizes Your Son's death and resurrection as we partake in Holy Communion. Lord, in our attempts to understand the mysteries of life, You gave us parables and sayings that connect heavenly messages with our frail human thinking. And so, You gave us the visions of one trying to make the new work by combining it with or pouring it into the old. This word tells us that sometimes, it is best to start anew. That lets us know there are second chances; that we cannot always expect to merely patch things up, but to let go, to find new vineyards, new wine, and new skins to hold our newness. Lord, as we help others, let us be grounded in the old; but we pray that You will also show us new ways to preserve the wine that comes at harvest time, and find new vessels, wineskins to contain our new bounty…

Change of View

VERSE FOR TODAY: Numbers 14:7-8

Joshua and Caleb said: "The land we passed through and explored is exceedingly good. If the LORD is pleased with us, he will lead us into that land, a land flowing with milk and honey, and will give it to us."

WE ALL PROBABLY remember this story that puts the Israelites on the brink of entering the Promised Land. They were poised to take possession of a land and settle down after escaping Pharaoh and leaving Egypt. They were finally moving toward their appointed destiny.

Moses was instructed to send 12 spies (one representing each of the tribes of Israel) to scout out the land of Canaan. The spies went on their journey assessing the land, the inhabitants, the fruit, the potential. They went eager and wide-eyed, curious, and intentional. They wanted to see if the people were "strong or weak, were they few or many, was the land good or bad, were the cities like camps or strongholds, was the land rich or poor, what about the forests?" (Numbers 13:28).

Twelve went, twelve took note, twelve made their reports. They did a **SWOT** Analysis. They formed their impressions of the **Strengths, Weaknesses, Opportunities, and Threats** of the Promised Land. They surveyed, they sampled, they marveled at the huge grapes. For 40 days, they conducted their analyses.

When it was time to present their findings, ten focused on the obstacles: giants, fortresses. Only these two, Joshua and Caleb, looked at the bounty: the milk and honey. For two, the taste of the grapes, pomegranates, figs, and faith in One who parted the Red Sea, produced manna and water, sent a cloud by day and a fire by night, formed their point of view. For ten, the giant descendants of Anak, the dwellers of the cities and the seaside, the stature of the men (humans) versus the status of God guided their view.

As helpers, our views determine our approach and expectations. We may often look at the obstacles and not the opportunities. We can be held captive by the policies, procedures, paperwork, bureaucracy, versus finding opportunities for creativity and a "can do" spirit to function within the boundaries. We often see the glass as half-empty, versus half-full; or we see the thorns and avoid picking the perfect bouquet of roses to lift someone's spirit.

Sometimes, as Joshua and Caleb, the only two adult Israelites to enter the Promised Land, we have to go with faith and conviction, viewing the strengths and opportunities as the action plan, rather than focusing on the weaknesses and threats. We even have to go on our convictions and go against the grain, as did Joshua and Caleb. Even when in the minority, we have to focus on the power of the positive, the possibilities not the problems.

NUGGET FOR TODAY: **I will focus on the milk and the honey, not the size of the problem.**

PRAYER FOR TODAY: Dear God of Manna and Quail, help us to remember that You will provide; that we are to simply go and possess the land. Forgive our grumbling; forgive our faintheartedness; forgive our desire to turn back, to take the easy road and turn back to Pharaoh. Forgive our tendency to focus on the problem, to see the thorn bushes, not the pomegranates and the figs. Forgive us for not seeing the milk and honey because we are focusing on the fortresses, the size of the people, not the size of You, our God. Help us to guide those we help to reach among the thorns and find the roses; help us to find vases and glass jars to display Your beautiful creations, serving as living testaments to Your goodness. Help us to focus on the possibilities, not the problems...

Fork in the Road

VERSE FOR TODAY: Matthew 7:13

Enter through the narrow gate. For wide is the gate and broad is the road that leads to destruction, and many enter through it. But small is the gate and narrow the road that leads to life, and only a few find it.

THE ROAD LESS traveled is a common phrase and the title of a book by M. Scott Peck. A fork in the road is perhaps an even more common reference to traveling. As I travel through towns and small cities, one of the best ways to avoid getting lost is to ask the locals for directions. When giving directions to my home in Midland, the less traveled outskirts of Columbus, Georgia, I would say, "When you come to a fork in the road, veer right." Just recently, as I needed directions, my host said, "Stay on Route 22 until you come to a fork in the road. Keep to the right until you see the Post Office, otherwise you'll end up crossing the railroad tracks and .... " Well, I didn't want to cross the tracks, so I wrote in big letters on my note pad: **VEER RIGHT**.

However, with improved signage, online maps, GPS (Global Positioning Systems), I find that people including myself still get lost. My friend gave me clear directions about what to do when I came to the fork in the road. Jesus also gives clear instructions, ones from the Great Navigator-God. Jesus instructs us to take the narrow gate-few will take the narrow way. So when you need to make a decision, don't follow the crowd.

Who knows what you will find when you take the narrow way? Though difficult to do when the world says get on the bandwagon, you may find...

- **Some rest spots...**
- **Some quiet places...**
- **Some park benches...**
- **Some cool water fountains...**
- **Some unique species of fawn and fauna...**

- **Some clear direction…**
- **Some new insights…**
- **Some clarity of vision…**
- **Some unexpected path to health, healing, and wholeness**.

Don't be tempted to follow the lure of the neon lights, beckoning and drawing you into their entanglements of busyness and distractions, even unethical behavior. The workplace has become a place that lacks integrity and ethics. It's gotten so bad that most helping disciplines require courses and continuing education workshops on ethics; many have to take out malpractice insurance. Some operate on an "if I can get away with it, do it attitude."

I encourage you to take the narrow way when tempted to sign in at the starting time even when you came in late. I encourage you to avoid whiling away the time you are paid by extending breaks or lunch hours. When tempted to pad the expense report, or when tempted to say you were on a field visit when you went shopping instead, take the narrow road. Even if you think you can get away with it, or "everybody's doing it," or the company has plenty of money, think of the fork in the road directions. Veer to the **RIGHT**. Who knows what may be **RIGHT** around the corner? The newspapers are full of stories of persons who thought no one would find out.

NUGGET FOR TODAY: I will follow the narrow path and veer RIGHT.

PRAYER FOR TODAY: Lord, the journey is filled with forks in the road and signs saying, "go this way," "go that way." Help us to focus on the narrow way, the way that leads to You. Help us to steer clear of thinking that no one will know, for we can't escape from Your presence and Your judgment. There are many decisions to be made in life, but veering to the **RIGHT**, Your way, will always keep us on the straight and narrow path. Help us to eliminate phrases like "everyone's doing it," for You call us to separate from the ways of the world that lead to destruction. There are few who find the narrow way; help us to be ever attentive to the signs saying veer to the **RIGHT,** that You post along the way…

Glory View

VERSE FOR TODAY: Isaiah 6:1

In the year that King Uzziah died, I saw the LORD sitting on a throne, high and exalted, and the train of his robe filled the temple.

ISAIAH AS WELL as Moses only got a glimpse of God's glory, since no man can see God and live. One of the attributes of God is that He is Spirit. He is personal—God is a living, speaking, feeling God.

Even though God told Moses that no one could see Him and live, God loves to come to us in ways that show His glory. He desires worship from us; and He desires to be gracious and compassionate to us. God has revealed Himself to earthly beings in many relationships, such as a Shepherd (Psalm 23), Provider (Matthew 6: 25, 33), Teacher (Psalm 25: 8-12), Counselor (Isaiah 9:6), and Friend (John 15:14-15).

God wants to show His glory by being intimately involved with His creations. Moses worshiped God after his encounter. Isaiah cried out "Woe is me for I am undone" (Isaiah 6:5). Isaiah realized he was a sinner and that he dwelt among sinners.

Surely Isaiah had entered the temple numerous times before. After the death of his believed to be cousin, King Uzziah, he may have had a different perspective, a mourning countenance that made him want to assess his life in God and his human frailty in light of death and eternity. He knew he was not capable of standing before God, so his whole view changed after this encounter. God's glory covered the temple; the Seraphim proclaimed the holiness of God. Isaiah knew this was no ordinary encounter—the earth was full of God's glory. King Uzziah was an earthly king, returned to the dust; but Isaiah had experienced the King of Kings; his view changed.

Isaiah's glory view experience of the Most High God, and the touch of hot coals on his lips made Isaiah's mission clear. When asked "whom shall I send?" without hesitation or reservation, Isaiah proclaimed: "Here am I, send me"(Isaiah 6:8). Isaiah knew he had a new job description: to describe and proclaim the experience of his "glory view."

When did you answer the call to be a helper? Did you sense a divine call? Did you experience God's glory? Were your lips touched by burning coals? Did you feel a fire deep within your spirit? Did you bow down in worship as Moses, or did you run from the call like Jonah? Did you get a glory view as you were mourning a loss of an earthly friend? Were you touched by homelessness, loneliness, hopelessness, hunger, mental and physical illness that made you cry out: "Here am I send me?" (Isaiah 6:8). Did you see an injustice and spring into action, crying out "woe is me?" (Isaiah 6:5). Did you become undone, grievous, because you suddenly had a glory view?

As Isaiah's glory view suddenly set him on a new path, did you also cry out send me…to the inner city, to the ghettos, to the psychiatric wards, to the homeless shelters, to the child welfare agencies, to juvenile justice facilities, to the foster homes, to the hospital, to the schools, to the hospices, to the clinics, to the jails, to the bedside…. to share this GLORY VIEW?

NUGGET FOR TODAY: I will answer, "Here am I, send me and I will go with confidence in the work I am being called to do.

PRAYER FOR TODAY: Lord, thank You for Isaiah's glory view. May we <u>not</u> be content until we have seen a glimpse of Your glory. May we hold Your glory sacred and may we share that view with others as we accept the call and answer: "Here we are, send us." Equip us to do Your work, let us bow down in reverence of Your glory that fills the temple; let us <u>not</u> run away like Jonah, feeling Your people are unworthy. May we fight for the less fortunate, play a small role in healing the land. Help us to become undone when we encounter injustices and say "We are people of unclean lips and we live among a people of unclean lips." Let us be like Isaiah, let us be cleansed, consecrated, and commissioned to help others have the joy of experiencing Your Glory View…

RSVP ASAP

Verse for Today: Luke 14:13

But, when you give a banquet, invite the poor, crippled, the lame, the blind, and you will be blessed. Although they cannot repay you, you will be repaid at the resurrection of the righteous.

We all know these familiar acronyms: RSVP (repondez, s'il vous plait)—please respond to the invitation, ASAP (as soon as possible). The first communicates a courtesy, the second a sense of urgency.

Think back. When was the last time you planned an event—a party, wedding, baby shower, cookout, luncheon? After deciding on the date, time, location, the next or perhaps the first task was to make up the guest list. Who do you want to honor *you* with *their* presence at *your* affair? When working as a bridal consultant, one of the most stressful and frustrating things was always the guest list. Who to invite, who to leave out, who is likely to come, in other words, who deserves an invitation? Are guests invited because of their *presence* or potential *presents*?

Our guest lists would probably include those from the previous verse in this parable, Verse 12—"friends, brothers or relatives, or your rich neighbors," lest they invite you back and the continuous social circle cycle happens—you invite them, they come, they invite you back; obligations abound. After all, we want to be on the list—and before we know it; our list expands.

Who would host a luncheon and invite the poor, blind, widowed, lonely, maimed, rather those who are not likely to pay us back? True hospitality, true service is manifested in how we treat those who can't repay, or so I thought. The team that traveled to West Africa went in sevice, expecting no repayment. The people openly welcomed and thanked us. They had little, but having hospitable spirits, they nonetheless, gave of their little, gave us gifts and fruit and smiles to say thank you—they gave us enduring memories.

So, as we think about ways to extend God's hospitality, how do helpers make up a guest list? Would we invite the ex-combatants who wreaked havoc on their own people, leaving many maimed, widowed, orphaned, during civil wars in West Africa, as did Rev. Herbert Zigbuo in Liberia, who led them in daily devotions? Would we invite the 16-year old boy who lost both arms to the rebels? Or, would we invite those who make us feel good by attending our affair and gracing us with their presence? Would we only invite those who could repay us with an even bigger party?

Helpers' guest lists must especially include those who are "cast offs" by society. Inviting them however, may be our greatest blessing. They provide us with opportunities to show God's love, to demonstrate God's concern for the poor and the outcasts. So, extend the invitation, expect a RSVP, and do it ASAP! It's urgent that we prepare a banquet for those who never receive an invitation.

NUGGET FOR TODAY: I will extend an invitation to those in need, expecting an RSVP ASAP.

Prayer for Today: Dear Lord of the Banquet, the One who has a feast waiting to repay the righteous at the resurrection, we pray that we will find many opportunities to extend an invitation to those that seldom receive them. Help us to <u>not</u> be so consumed by who can grace us by their appearance at our banquets, but to be consumed with planning a party for those who never appear on high society guest lists. Lord, we know many people select their guest lists by inviting those who can repay them, or can enlarge their social circle, or can make them look good, or provide the best food, drink, and desserts. Lord, we just want to invite people who can feast on You, drink of Your Healing Water, taste the sweetness of Your Spirit so that the places of honor will be to spend time in Your presence. As helpers, may we RSVP to Your example of who should make up the guest list. Help us to do this ASAP…

Emergency Preparedness

VERSE FOR TODAY: Matthew 25:13

Therefore keep watch, because you do not know the day or the hour.

SINCE RECENT MAN-MADE disasters like 9/11, and natural disasters like tsunamis, floods, fires, mudslides, earthquakes, hurricanes such as Katrina and Rita, since a Midwestern blackout, everyone is talking about emergency preparedness. Municipalities have developed response teams and escape plans; families and individuals have developed emergency evacuation plans. Lists from the Red Cross advise us of things to keep handy: flashlights, candles, generators, bottled water, first aid kits, even chewing gum, and garbage bags. Everyone is being cautioned to develop a plan of escape in case of an emergency.

Can we really be prepared? At least we like to hope so. We don't want to be like the "five foolish virgins" in our passage today. In total, ten virgins were waiting for the bridegroom. The text tells us that five of the virgins were waiting for the bridegroom, but took no oil for their lamps. They ran out of oil before the bridegroom came. They asked the other five who had oil to share theirs, but they refused to share. Then the oil-less five went to buy oil only to find the bridegroom had come while they were gone.

Just like these five "foolish virgins," so many of us will find ourselves unprepared in the event of an emergency. We will have lamps with no oil, cars with no gas, flashlights with no batteries, candles with no matches—useless in an emergency. We stock up and prepare after an emergency, only to become lax after danger has passed. So what does this tell us? It reminds me of a Negro Spiritual: *Keep your lamps trimmed and burning.*

The five foolish virgins lacked wisdom or "oil for their lamps." So, as we help others we must keep oil in our lamps and keep the wicks trimmed by cutting off the charred ends, thus enabling the lamps to burn the oil.

We do not know when a disaster may strike, and we also don't know when an opportunity may come our way. Therefore, it is wise to help those we help to be prepared for the worst, as well as the unexpected in the form of positive things. It's wise to have a backup plan, wise to have an escape plan, wise to do a dry run to be ever ready. What if a client were starting a new job on Monday? Is there a backup plan in case he/she misses the bus? How will he/she know how long the trip to work takes without a dry run? How will he/she extricate him or herself from a situation that may threaten a new job? What if the babysitter changes her mind or a child gets sick? How will clients be prepared to take on a new opportunity if they have not "trimmed their wicks" with discipline, training, education, job skills, and making dry runs?

NUGGET FOR TODAY: I will be prepared for unexpected challenges and opportunities.

PRAYER FOR TODAY: Lord, You are the Bridegroom. You can come at any time. You can present us with a challenge or an opportunity at any time. We pray that we will take emergency preparedness seriously. We want to keep oil for our lamps; we want to keep the wicks trimmed; we never know when batteries may need charging or electricity may go out. We want to be awake and energized to face what each day brings. We pray that we will not depend on buying oil from others, but keep back-up oil if needed. We pray for an escape route from all that might hinder or deter us from escaping the tsunamis and mudslides of life that may come. Most of all, we want to be ready when You come, because You clearly state in today's verse that no one knows the day or the hour…

Plowing Time

VERSE FOR TODAY: Luke 9:62

Jesus replied, "No one who puts his hand to the plow and looks back is fit for service in the kingdom of God."

PLOWING. WHETHER PLOWING with oxen, mules, horses, or tractors, it is hard to plow while looking back. I remember how my father and his farming friends and our neighbors prided themselves on straight rows in their gardens. Meticulous rows were the sign of one focused on the task, a master plower and gardener. In the verse for today, Jesus gives a lesson on the need to focus on God. Plowing is serious business.

Jesus uses the analogy of plowing. Plowing rows and furrows in preparation for planting provides a lesson for everyday life. Last Sunday, I traveled through parts of rural Ohio, just as corn plants were beginning to show their heads. It was easy to see the neat rows that went on and on for miles and miles, acres and acres, farm to farm. This was the optimal time to see the neat rows. Once the corn becomes full grown, it's difficult to distinguish the rows.

One of my favorite annual activities is to go to the Ohio State Fair and marvel at the huge farming equipment that now does the work I remember being done by men and horses. The animal and the plower work in tandem. The animal pulls, the plower guides. If the plower becomes distracted, even for a second, there goes the neat row. So it's hard to plow when distracted and impossible when looking back even with million dollar modern day machinery.

After my father plowed neat orderly rows at the right width and depth for the particular seed, we children carefully sprinkled or placed the seeds, a bit of fertilizer, a cup of water in the furrow, covered the seeds and waited for the pay-off. Sprouts, then fruit, then harvest time. In all of the mystery of harvest time, it was important to focus on the yield and not look back. We didn't want to pull up the plants before they had produced their fruit.

So as helpers work with clients, patients, students, parishioners, and those needing care, it is important to help them focus on what is ahead. No one can focus on the future while constantly looking back on the past. Keeping focused on a goal or task, putting a hand to the plow, trusting in God to bring the increase is the formula for hitting the mark—the kingdom of God. As Lot's wife turned to a pillar of salt (Genesis 19:6), that can be our fate if we focus on looking back, if we focus on what was or might have been rather than on the neat, fertile furrows of a newly plowed field of opportunity.

NUGGET FOR TODAY: I will plow straight furrows, by focusing on what's ahead.

PRAYER FOR TODAY: Dear Lord of the Harvest, You teach us to focus on You. How can we keep our hands on the plow and not look back? In our human tendencies, we are often like Lot's wife. We may cling to the comfort of what's behind rather than plowing ahead to greener pastures, fertile ground, a harvest of blessings. Help us to stay focused on You. We want to be fit for the kingdom. As You pull us along, let us guide the plow toward the vast acres of bounty awaiting those who stay focused on You. We will keep our hands on the plow, focusing on You, what lies ahead, what You have planned for us, and the work You have designated as we help others...

Seed-Lings

VERSE FOR TODAY: Matthew 13:31-32

He told them another parable: "The kingdom of heaven is like a mustard seed, which a man took and planted in his field. Though it is the smallest of all your seeds, yet when it grows, it is the largest of garden plants and becomes a tree, so that the birds of the air come and perch in its branches."

SOMETIMES, YOU JUST can't tell.

The mustard seed is small indeed—so what type of tree can it become? The tree will be much larger than the seed seems to predict. Mustard trees grow to about ten feet tall. So, even though small, the seed can produce a tree of height and breadth, providing a place for birds to perch.

One year during installation of officers for our women's mission group, I gave each of the women a seed. They tried to guess what each seed was. To the unseasoned eye, it's hard to know what a seed is. Is it a ...

Marigold
Turnip (so small, it is hard to keep from losing it)
Delphinium
Petunia
Geranium
Daisy
Sunflower (we may be familiar with sunflower seeds from feeding the birds)?

Or is it an...
Annual
Perennial
Biennial?

What about the seeds of the great conifers?
Is it a ...
Pinecone for a pine tree
Or will it be a giant redwood tree?

From this teaching of Jesus, we learn that even though we may have a small beginning, we have great possibilities. Even though we have little to start, we can become prosperous. This is a great lesson to share with those we help. The starting point does not determine the destiny. Encourage those we serve to plant whatever seeds they have, knowing God sees great growth opportunities for every seedling.

NUGGET FOR TODAY: Today I will plant seeds of hope.

PRAYER FOR TODAY: Dear God of Great Possibilities, You made every seed uniquely equipped to reproduce itself. The marigold does not become a petunia; the apple seed does not produce peaches; the turnip seed does not produce eggplants. How amazing is the study of seeds. How gratifying it is to know that the size of the seed does not determine the size of the plant. A mustard seed produces a great tree and shares its branches with the birds of the air. Thank You God that each seed has the potential to produce bountiful results. Help us to nurture our seed-LINGS. Help us to plant seeds of hope, knowing that the right combination of sun and water that You provide will lead to a bountiful harvest...

I ~~Messed~~ Up!

VERSE FOR TODAY: Lamentations 3:22-23

Because of the LORD's great love, we are not consumed, for his compassions never fail. They are new every morning; great is thy faithfulness.

THESE VERSES FORM the basis for one of my favorite hymns, *Great is Thy Faithfulness.* This new opportunity every morning reminds me of one of the youth in our church. During the annual Christmas and Easter cantatas, the young people in our church are invited to participate, usually by singing solos related to the music and narration of the cantata.

One Christmas, a young lady was singing to a full audience surrounded by all the decorations and excitement of a major production when stage fright overcame her. She suddenly went blank. She said "Oops! I messed up" and asked the director: "Can I start over?" The caring and concerned director nodded "yes," and to everyone's delight, the young lady began over and sang with fervor and conviction. The second start was so powerful that no one thought much about the earlier pronouncement: "I messed up."

This verse points to God's faithfulness. He knows we will mess up, but gives the assurance that He will continue to remain faithful and allow us to start over. He believes in second chances and looks for repentant souls and well-meaning helpers to simply say: "I messed up." I completed the wrong paperwork, I made the wrong diagnosis, *I "coulda, woulda, shoulda."* Although our mistakes can have devastating effects on those we serve, God surrounds us with protection, love, mercy, and discipline, when we mess up despite our best intentions.

This faithfulness and chance to start over again is also available to those we serve. Yes, they got off the diet, yes they started smoking, drinking, using, abusing again. It's important to help those we serve and care for to gain the confidence and discipline to begin again, to incrementally extinguish those self-defeating habits, those actions that took place today. Because, tomorrow holds new mercies, a new opportunity to not be consumed, a new opportunity to celebrate that our transgressions are removed as far as the "east is from the west" (Psalm 103:12). We are not consumed; the comforting, compassionate character of God says there is no situation that we don't have a chance to confess, "I messed up" and petition by asking, "Can I start over?" We should be as honest as this young child to realize when we need to start over assured by God's grace, mercy, and faithfulness.

For helpers, it is important to help those we help who may backslide or "mess up," to let go of the burdens of a single incident or even a lifetime of messing up. God has made it clear that He understands that we mess up. So, let's help clients to fess up and move on.

Nugget for Today: If I mess up, I can start again.

Prayer for Today: Dear God of Second Chances, where would we be without Your forgiveness and Your grace? Your Word says Your compassions never fail; we receive new mercies every morning, and You are faithful to forgive us when we mess up. Lord, as hard as we try sometimes, it seems we just don't quite get it right. We get off to a bad start; we let one transgression mount up to become a mountain of things we know we should not be doing. So Lord, we will do our best not to mess up, but when we do, we will fess up and hold You to Your promise of faithfulness, grace, and forgiveness. Yes, each day is a new opportunity and we want to focus on getting it right, to avoid constantly having to start over. Help us to help guide those we serve to have this same conviction and determination...

In-Di-Gestion

VERSE FOR TODAY: Romans 14:23

But the man who has doubts is condemned if he eats, because his eating is not from faith; and everything that does not come from faith is sin.

THERE CAN BE many versions of the familiar saying: "You are what you eat." For example: you are what you believe; or you are what you think are further references to some status being the result of some mental action. This passage combines the verb phrase *you are* .... with two nouns "doubt" and "faith." But, when I first read this passage, I asked myself: "What does this have to do with eating?" Well, can it be that if we doubt, it's no use eating, I ask? If we doubt, when we eat will we get full? Maybe we shouldn't eat at all. This could be a good new diet craze. Or, if we eat without faith, will the food get stuck in our being, causing in-di-gestion? You may as well get the purple pill or the Alka Seltzer™ because doubt is obviously hard to digest. Doubt chokes out faith; doubt leads to condemnation.

Earlier, in this chapter (Romans 14:21), we were also admonished not to eat meat or drink wine if it causes our brother to fall or stumble. When preparing the buffet, we must carefully select the offerings—will the meat cause someone to stumble, choke, or to doubt; will the wine cause someone to stumble, choke, doubt? If we feast on doubt and leave faith off the menu, we can get a serious bout of in-di-gestion because we will ultimately engage in sin which should be hard to swallow.

It is important then as helpers, that we help those we care for to avoid in-di-gestion with a well-rounded menu of healthy foods, with adequate portions, and daily servings of faith. We must help them make healthy eating and living choices, avoiding things that choke them, things that cause doubt. A heaping of faith, goes a long way because faith can move mountains, make our works come to life, and cure in-di-gestion.

NUGGET FOR TODAY: **I am what I eat, believe and think. Today I will select adequate servings from the menu of faith.**

PRAYER FOR TODAY: Dear Lord and Provider of every good and perfect thing, we pray that we will be selective in our diet. Lord, we want to choose those things that will give us faith, give us strength, and cure in-di-gestion caused by eating foods that choke us and bring about doubt. We know that what we take in becomes part of us, so help us to in-gest wholesome, filling, affirming morsels. We are what we eat, so we want to feast on You and Your goodness, Your provision, Your faithfulness, and Your desire for us is to be well-nourished and productive. We thank You for condemning the sin caused by doubt and we will endeavor this and every day to feast on Your bounty, praying for faith, positive beliefs, and positive thoughts...

Get on First

Verse for Today: Mark 4:28

All by itself the crop produces grain—first the stalk, then the head, then the full kernel in the head.

An earlier verse in this parable of the growing seed (Verse 26) indicates that the farmer sows the seed but does not know how the seed grows. Even with the latest technology and equipment, man does not know how seeds grow. Yes, you say we know that water and light are ingredients that make plants grow. We know about photosynthesis. We have developed hydroponics—growing plants in water or solutions, and we've developed hybrids, and new cultivars. Even so we can only plant and expect or hope our seeds will grow.

This parable points to orderliness and sequential steps. First the sowing, then the stalk appears, then the full head, and finally the grain that can be harvested to produce seeds for the next harvest. Or, the seed, then the bud, then the flower, or the seedling, then the tree, then the fruit. First things first.

Children are always amazed at growing seeds. When the first sprout appears, their excitement explodes. The sprout is only the beginning of the process; the real excitement comes when we can actually harvest our seeds, pick the tomatoes, smell the flowers, eat the apple.

Man also recognizes the importance of process, structure and orderliness. We know one has to crawl before one can walk; or one must eat soft food before eating a pork chop. One must put the horse before the cart if the horse is to pull the load.

What about America's favorite pastime, baseball? Even though a batter hits a grand slam home run with the bases loaded, every runner must touch first base and round all the bases before touching home. Failure to touch any of the bases or home plate will result in a call of **"You're OUT!**

So often the helper has to understand the importance of first things first, baby steps. The issues and problems of those we help did not just occur overnight; thus solutions must be orderly with first things first. Just as a baby learning to walk falls down and has setbacks, so too must helpers understand and even to some extent, anticipate some falling down.

When students in my classes, research classes especially, get the syllabi for the semester, they invariably begin to stress over the final assignment. If I were conducting a research study of that, I could easily count the number of times this happens. Once the stress comes to a crescendo, I then say, "The final assignment builds on everything that takes place before it. The lectures, readings, discussions, and other assignments are the baby steps that lead to a full understanding of the final assignment."

So too in life, the assignments build upon each other, just as the blade, head, full grain, then the harvest. As with baseball, if the runner gets stuck on third, that doesn't count. Rounding all the bases is the only way to score. First things first.

NUGGET FOR TODAY: Today, I will round the bases by touching first, then moving to second, third, and finally touching home.

PRAYER FOR TODAY: Loving Father, Author of Orderliness, help us find comfort in the fact that whatever we do will be better if we utilize some sense of purpose, orderliness, and planning. Help us to understand that even with a home run, we have to touch first base first. When planting seeds of hope in those we help, help us to begin where they are; we have to help them take baby steps, moving forward one step at a time. Help us to also understand that sometimes, they will fall down, so we pray that we can help them get up and start over again. Help us to understand that new methods such as hydroponics for plants may help clients to reach their goals, but ultimately for them, and us, You give the increase; You help the plants to grow and the cycle of life is determined by You. We want to be faithful planters and good harvesters, realizing that it is necessary to put You in front of the cart, because putting the cart before the horse will be useless. We want to get on first...

Only is Lonely

Two are better than one, because they have a good return for their work: If one falls down, his friend can help him up. But pity the man who falls and has no one to help him up!

Many illustrations point to the benefit of togetherness, the value of a friend, trusted companion, or confidant. Friends bring intimacy, sharing, comfort, and defense. Friends help one to think things through—"two heads are better than one." A Chinese proverb that I learned years back indicates, "many hands make light work."

Two illustrations point to the value of companionship. Whenever I cook out and use charcoal, I am reminded of a picture painted by a former pastor—if a glowing log or charcoal is taken from the fire and left by itself, it will soon go out. It needs the heat and warmth of other briquettes and logs to burn its best, to burn to completion.

Ecclesiastes 4:11 provides a human illustration of this phenomenon: "Also, if two lie down together, they will keep warm, but how can one keep warm alone?" Yes, we need each other. The warmth from two bodies together provides the "synergy" to keep them both warm. Likewise, if two combine forces against an enemy they are more likely to prevail. Or a "threefold cord", wound tightly is less likely to break even though it may fray. Ecclesiastes 4:12 states: "A cord of three strands is not quickly broken."

On special occasions like Mother's Day and Christmas, I often think of the lonely—those who have no one to brighten their day with a card, phone call, or a message of cheer. No one to visit them in the hospital, halfway house, juvenile detention center, residential treatment center, or nursing home; no one to pin a flower on them or give them a present, not even anyone to give them a hug. The saddest of all—no one to pray for them. Only is lonely.

Jesus even discussed the meaningfulness of two in Matthew Chapter 18 verses 19-20 regarding two who agree. He gives us assurance that when two agree, they can ask for anything and it will be given; or where two or three are gathered together in His name, He will be in the midst.

NUGGET FOR TODAY: I will try to find special, supportive companions to share the journey with me.

PRAYER FOR TODAY: Lord, You made us for companionship. Even You, the Creator of the Universe, felt the need for someone when You stated in the Beginning that You were lonely. Thus You created us mere mortals for companions for You and each other. Then after You created the first human, Adam, You knew he would be lonely in that special place You made for man; so You uniquely fashioned a companion, helper for him—someone to talk to, to tell his troubles to, someone to help bear the load. And just as with Your first humans, we need someone to lean on, someone to keep the fire lit, someone to help keep us warm. We know the warmth of Your love is there for us, but human companionship helps us along the journey. Lord, help us to be a threefold cord. Help us to wind ourselves tightly with love and friendship so that we will form a bond that is not easily broken. Lord, we know that the ends of friendship may become tattered and frayed as with a cord. As helpers and caregivers we know that those we help will often find themselves dealing with problems and weaknesses by themselves. But You are the glue that holds us together. May we find strength, support, and sustenance in our earthly companions. Help us to keep each other warm...

Jig Saw Puzzle

VERSE FOR TODAY: Judges 21:3

"O LORD, the God of Israel," they cried, "why has this happened to Israel? Why should one tribe be missing from Israel today?"

HAVE YOU EVER seen a beautiful mosaic, or a tapestry, or a tile floor with a piece missing? For a mosaic the beauty is impaired. For a tapestry one missing thread could cause the entire weaving to unravel. For a missing tile, a person could trip. Think about a young child with a most beautiful smile. The missing front tooth captures our attention and often focuses the conversation on the one missing tooth, rather than those still remaining.

During our annual women's School of Mission, in the time set aside for quiet reflection, the women spend hours putting together jig saw puzzles, focusing on the beautiful picture on the box as a guide. Different women come by, add to the puzzle, and usually by week's end, the puzzle is complete. But just imagine how these women would feel if they put 999 pieces together only to find one missing. I suspect they would be really disappointed despite the joint effort of everyone. But, it is also important to know that sometimes one doesn't know what's missing until the puzzle is finished.

Today's verse from Judges talks about the defeat of the Benjamites. After a great military defeat, the remaining tribes of Israel felt this entire tribe would be wiped out and therefore, they engaged in a brutal and questionable campaign to get wives for the single Benjamite men to make sure this tribe would not be missing from their ranks. Marrying these women from other nations ultimately caused "everyone to do what was right in his own eyes" (Judges 21:25), forgetting their promises and trust in God.

By focusing on the missing tribe, the morals of everyone became diluted. Helpers should help clients, patients, and those we serve and care for to be aware of what may be missing, but we should refrain from focusing all of the attention and energy on the missing element. Instead, let's help those we care for to see the beauty of the whole puzzle, the 999 pieces and as a result, let's find ways to supplant or overcome the missing pieces. It is important to see the beauty of the whole puzzle even though not perfect, rather than making the missing piece the central focus. Let us not try to supplant the missing with unhealthy, unwholesome activities and things.

NUGGET FOR TODAY: I will focus on the beauty of the whole puzzle rather than spend time and energy seeing only the missing piece.

PRAYER FOR TODAY: Lord, You created beautiful and magnificent things. You also gave us talents and skills to make beautiful creations. You gave us the gift of quiet time or private time to play games, to put puzzles together, and to find distractions from our work. But Lord, often we miss the beauty of the whole puzzle, because we can't seem to move past the missing pieces. Yes, sometimes we don't realize what's missing until we put the whole puzzle together. How like helpers to spend so much time helping to put the pieces together only to find that someone has made off with a crucial piece. But Lord, help us to not despair. Help us to avoid extreme measures, but rather help us to find meaningful, effective ways to fill in what may be missing...

Savings Account

VERSE FOR TODAY: Romans 10:9

That if you confess with your mouth, "Jesus is Lord." and believe in your heart that God raised him from the dead, you will be saved.

CONFESSING, BELIEVING, CALLING on the Lord for help is easy and for many, even automatic when we're in a foxhole situation with enemy fire all about. Some times we are so casual about using God in a sentence, "O my god," that I'm convinced that few may realize they are taking "God's" name in vain. With such demonstrations of pleasure, pride, even joy—there is a strong possibility that the speaker is not really thinking of the One who makes all things happen.

Confessing that Jesus is Lord and that He was raised from the dead are the only deposits needed for the bank account of eternal life. No matter the order, confess/believe, believe/ confess interest in the account of salvation will accumulate. The one who believes will not be put to shame—no there are no restrictions on who can open an account—Jew or Greek (Romans 10:11, 10:12).

We often tell those we help to "confess", come clean, and admit to veering from the goals and the treatment plan. Confession is good for the soul. Coming clean is a first step towards recovery. We all know when we've had one drink too many, one high too many, one candy bar or piece of cheesecake too many. It's important to urge our clients to begin to make come clean deposits beginning with confession. Drug tests are revealing, but confessing and admitting to our transgressions lead to healing and wholeness. But, more importantly, the confession account leads to eternal salvation. By believing and confessing the risen Christ, the account can be opened at any time; deposits can be made at any time; and best of all the interest and dividends of believing lead to eternal rewards.

101 Helps for Helpers

Nugget for Today: I will open up my account by simply saying "Jesus is Lord."

Prayer for Today: Lord, You made it so simple; You simply said confess and believe. We will strive to do both of these as we make deposits to our eternal bank accounts. We know these daily deposits will reap great returns. We spend time and energy on earthly accounts, saving for worldly, temporal things; we want to move beyond the here and now. We want more than savings; **we want to be saved…**

Mountain Marvels

Verse for Today: Matthew 17:20

He replied, "Because you have so little faith, I tell you the truth, if you have faith as small as a mustard seed, you can say to this mountain, 'Move from here to there' and it will move. Nothing will be impossible for you."

Mountains always amaze me. Growing up in Georgia, I barely got a glimpse or understanding of mountains except the famous Stone Mountain near Atlanta with the carvings of Civil War figures. Later, I had the opportunity to glimpse Mt. Rushmore, Mt. Rainier, and mountains in Yosemite and other national parks and the Sierra Nevada mountains. None however was as magnificent as the Alps Mountains, which cover a considerable portion of the landscape of Europe, fashioning much of the culture and activities.

As a child, I thought mountains were made of compacted earth. But lessons in geology and personal enlightenment made mountains even more awesome. Viewing the Alps Mountain from an airplane, on the ground or from a hotel room reveal the unimaginable size, splendor and endurance of mountains. So to think that mustard seed faith can move gargantuan mountains warrants attention and action. This exhibition of faith is all that's needed.

While looking out the plane window on a return trip from Rome, Italy after an overnight delay in Milan, Italy, the pilot needed to change course and tipped the plane's wings toward the Alps Mountains below. How majestic! I just thought if a small seed of faith can move any one of the peaks that seemed to go on forever, surely I could muster up faith as large as a **Georgia peach seed**.

So, helpers let's start collecting seeds. Let's move some mountains; let's see how we can help those we help to fling mountains of poverty, addiction, lack of education, homelessness, illiteracy, disease, hunger, unemployment, mental illness, delinquency, despair, apathy, hopelessness ….into the sea. The power is there; just plant the seeds of faith.

Little seed, large mountain
Little faith, large GOD.

NUGGET FOR TODAY: I will plant mountain-moving seeds of hope and expectation this day.

PRAYER FOR TODAY: Dear Mountain Moving God, You made it clear— faith is the answer. Just the faith of a mustard seed, can sprout into mountain-moving marvels. Mountains can be flung into the sea if we would just plant the faith seeds. Faith can seep through the crevices, sprout on the landings, burst forth on the summit if we would just plant the seeds. Lord, You gave us an arsenal of mountain-moving seeds when You led us to choose helping others. You gave us the fertile soil to plant them in. As we help others to till the soil, sow the seeds, and reap the harvest, we know that no mountain can stand between You, the Rock, and the blessings You have for those who have the faith. So we go forth today with the assurance that we can achieve the impossible with mustard seed faith...

It's Okay to RE-treat

Verse for Today: Jeremiah 6:16

This is what the Lord says: "Stand at the crossroads and look; ask for the ancient paths, ask where the good way is, and walk in it, and you will find rest for your souls."

Jeremiah is known as the "weeping prophet." Beset with anguish and turmoil, he struggled with the message of judgment he was called to prophesy about-drought, famine, sword (Chapter 14). He suffered many hardships, including being thrown into a well because of his message. But, he had a fire within his bones that made him steadfast in what God told him to do.

Jeremiah encouraged the people to remember the traditions, triumphs, and wonders of God from the past. He was advising them to retreat, turn back to the former days spent in worship and devotion. The sad part of this story is that the people refused to **RE…**

RE-member-the tried and true ways

RE-flect and contemplate the past

RE-treat to former ways so that they might find rest from their wanderings into sin. They continued in their sinful ways declaring: "We will not walk in it" (Verse 16).

The sound of the trumpet should have been a wake-up call but—refusing to **RE**-treat led to calamity.

RE-treating to old ways, remembering, standing at the crossroads, walking well-worn, familiar paths, **RE**-membering the old ways-where the good way is, this is the path to walk. A walk down memory lane is often good for the soul. It helps one to **RE**-treat to the safety of knowing that if you made it once, it's possible to do it again. **RE**-treating, taking time out is rest for the soul, because it helps us to **RE**-energize, **RE**-focus, **RE**-flect, and **RE**-pent.

RE-treating from a military standpoint is considered to be a sign of cowardice or weakness, but to **RE**-treat when the battle is too big, can lead to a sense of **RE**-assurance that can lead to obedience and rest, **RE**-considering if the battle were worth it in the first place. Yes, helping those we serve to **RE**-treat from actions that are self-destructive and **RE**-treat to the peace and rest available in finding and walking in the good way can lead to success, *REST*, and ultimately peace.

NUGGET FOR TODAY: **I will RE-treat to the places that I walked along the way, finding REST from the trials of the day.**

PRAYER FOR TODAY: Lord, help us to learn to RE-treat. We have walked along many paths, we have felt pain, and defeat as well as joy and triumph. Help us to walk again the ancient paths. Help us to ask and know where the "good way" is. Help us <u>not</u> be stubborn as the people in Jeremiah's days by refusing to walk in the "good way." Help us to stroll along this good path, savoring the memory of the good things and finding consolation for the things that did not go as expected. Help us to listen to the voices of those who want to direct us to the paths of RE-treat and let us bathe in the assurance that we can avoid the disaster brought on by the people in Jeremiah's day if we would RE-member to RE-treat…

Cruise Control

VERSE FOR TODAY: Romans 8:28

And we know that in all things God works for the good of those who love him, who have been called according to his purpose.

DURING DEVOTIONAL TIME in a meeting a few years ago, everyone was asked to share their favorite Bible verse and share why they chose that verse. Several persons lifted this verse and their rationale was the assurance that God was in control, that whatever one attempts will work out well if it is divinely ordained and divinely inspired, for a divine purpose.

Sometimes, we don't know what to do, what to ask, how to plan; when to say yes, when to say no; when to act, when to be still; when to be assertive, when to be passive; and how to work with different players at different times regarding different things. Trying to put all the pieces together into a master plan can be daunting, so much so that many never get far in their endeavors.

Reflecting on this passage reminds me of cars equipped with cruise control, a feature found on most cars nowadays. Set the speed, steer the vehicle, don't get too comfortable, though—especially in heavy traffic, rain, snow, or bad weather. So cruise control on a luxury car even with the latest equipment still requires some attention and action by the driver. When we engage the cruise control, we can focus on God, let God steer the wheel and set the course, knowing that the results will be favorable if ordained by Him.

Let go, Let God!—who causes all things to work together as He sets the cruising speed and steers the plan. As we develop treatment plans, let God put the pieces together—just trust Him for the outcome, believing we have been called to serve others for His purpose. What God desires to accomplish will work together for good for His human creations, for His divine purpose.

Sometimes the time and energy we spend to bring about a human-inspired outcome can be counterproductive to a God-inspired plan. Count on God to make things work to His glory. Continue to keep your eyes on the road, though trusting God to lead you toward His inspired destination.

NUGGET FOR TODAY: Today I will cruise with God in control.

PRAYER FOR TODAY: Dear God, You are omniscient, omnipresent and omnipotent. You know all things; You are everywhere; and You are all powerful. You control the universe. You micromanage the affairs of all creations, animate and inanimate. You control the comings and goings of the universe. There is nothing that happens that You don't know about or have Your hands in. So, God we will learn today to engage the cruise control with You at the steering wheel. Lord, we try so hard to make a difference in the lives of those we help and care for, but we are often at a loss for the best way to serve. So Lord, we rest in the promise of knowing that all things work together for good if we are called according to Your purpose. We will cruise with that assurance…

Almost, But!

VERSE FOR TODAY: Psalm 73:2

But as for me, my feet had almost slipped; I had nearly lost my foothold.

ALMOST…BUT!

ALMOST INDICATES NOT quite. I almost gave in. I almost stumbled. I almost got lost. I almost got that job. I almost won the lottery. I almost … Can you remember a time when you almost *did* something or almost *did not* do something?

When traveling to Mexico a couple summers ago, I got bold and adventurous. I decided to go for the thrill of riding on a banana boat. My sister and two nieces and I donned our life jackets and were pulled by a fast-moving boat out onto the open waters of the Sea of Cortèz.

I almost changed my mind, BUT…

Determined to hold on, ride the waves and scream my head off—I was the tourist extraordinaire. How about this for a vacation venture? Was anyone taking pictures for me to show off to the people back home? Until, that is the exciting ride became terrifying when I was thrown into the rough sea. Foolish me-I didn't even *quite* know how to swim.

I almost finished my swimming lessons, BUT…

I was struggling to keep afloat and keep my head above water…

I almost drowned, BUT…

I remember my sister's saying as long as you have a life jacket on you won't go under. She was referring to the man-made life jacket I was wearing. I needed the Divine Life Jacket to keep me afloat.

101 Helps for Helpers

I kept remembering her words, **but** I wasn't too sure about that until I was pulled, terrified and shaken onto the safety of the boat.

As I continue to reflect on that **almost** drowning experience, two things came to mind when I was safely on dry land. First, Love lifted me. I know God's Love saved me. Secondly, I also know that the Life Jacket saved me. Not the cheap plastic one provided by the boat company, but by the Life Jacket of the One who is the Master of the Sea, the One who commands the winds and waves to obey, the One who can hold you up during the fearsome waves. The One who lets your feet slip or your head go under, the One who won't let you perish. The One who always throws out a lifeline if one would just grab a hold.

Yes, Almost… BUT indicates that you may slip, but you don't have to fall.

As helpers struggle to help those we serve keep their heads above water when the bills are high and the funds are low, who help buffet them from being tossed to and fro when the storms of life are raging, who help give them an anchor against a callous society, who help those who are sinking deeper into depression and despair, who help those who are far from the shore of safety and security, who help those who can't bask in the radiance of the Mexican sun, who don't know the victory of the SON, who help those who are sinking to rise no more, may you be encouraged to say **almost…BUT**. Throw out a lifeline, pull them to safety, and help them to rest on the shore so that they can proclaim: I have made the Sovereign LORD my refuge.

Nugget for Today: Almost…BUT. Today I will trust in the Master of the Sea.

Prayer for Today: Dear Master of the Sea, the only One who can truly throw out the life line and rescue us, we thank You for safety when the storms of life are raging. Lord, give us an anchor to guide and lead us as we serve others, and also one for those in need of stability when being tossed and driven by the raging waters of life. Lord, we long for the peaceful shore where we can bask in the glow and warmth of the sun and Your Son, but sometimes, all we can do is keep our head above the water. We thank You that You are the Life Jacket that we can always count on to keep us afloat. In our humanness, enable us to help those we serve to be pulled safely to the shore. Lord we look for the many times when we can say with triumph…

We almost…BUT…

Foot on the Brake

VERSE FOR TODAY: Mark 16:15

He said to them: "Go into all the world and preach the good news to all creation."

THIS FAMILIAR SCRIPTURE is also known as a first component of the Great Commission. This charge is found in all four of the gospels. We all receive numerous calls to go—but often we put our foot on the brake.

When wheeled vehicles were invented, in addition to figuring out mechanisms to make them go, inventors or users had to also figure out how to make them stop—thus brakes. When I had the opportunity to travel to Sierra Leone and Liberia, West Africa some months ago, two things fascinated me. First, stop signs and traffic lights were virtually non-existent. However, people managed to maneuver the busy, crowded streets without causing major accidents or traffic jams.

Another thing that caught my attention was the many wheeled vehicles, rather wheeled, makeshift contraptions. Anything with wheels—baby strollers, wagons, carts, wheel barrows, creatively fashioned contraptions of all sorts, were useful for carting loads of fruit, vegetables, bottled water, Cokes and Fanta, firewood, charcoal, clothes, shoes, building materials, to sell to anyone—whatever could be used or sold. These vehicles used the braking power of humans when near collisions were imminent.

In addition, when I think about the fervor in which my only brother, Albert, Jr. embraced wheeled vehicles, I lovingly reflect on the numerous pairs of tennis shoes he wore out stopping a scooter, wagon, or some makeshift contraption he fashioned. He even stopped bikes with his feet. When I learned to ride a bike, brakes were on the pedal—pedal forward to go forth; press backward to stop. Now bikes have sophisticated hand brake systems. Automotive technology has outdone itself when it comes to brakes—hydraulics, anti-locking braking systems. Automotive technology is even trying to develop stabilization systems that can stop on ice. Imagine—that should go over well in the Cleveland, Ohio winters.

The challenge in this verse is to go—no braking needed. But, we tend to put our feet on the brake when it comes to spreading the Good News to others—we don't mind stop and go traffic then. We don't mind stop and go traffic when we are called to go to those undesirable places of our calling.

This brake phenomenon while driving is intriguing to say the least, and also aggravating. Have you ever noticed people who drive with their foot on the brake? Going along at a reasonable speed, even speeding up with their foot on the brake—brake lights on while traveling 40 mph is a good tip off. Or, what about the driver who drives at *break*neck speed during rush hour traffic, only to brake a few feet later. And then, there's the driver who brakes for no apparent reason (well you might conclude the cell phone rings, that has proven to be the case all too often lately). And again, the drivers who engage in random acts of braking. Are they indecisive, do they really want to reach their destination? Do they think about the adjustments the driver behind them has to make? Indecisive, in a hurry, distracted, unaware of the flow of traffic, these impact our driving braking habits.

Well, let's help clients move ahead freely, not with their foot on the brake, but going the speed limit, going with the flow of traffic. Let the helpers focus on the "go" command. Go without regard to race, gender, class, status of the person needing help. Let us not be like Jonah who thought he should decide who was worth helping and ended up in the belly of a whale. Stopping and going is a reality in rush-hour traffic, but let's go full speed ahead to the needy, lost, and dispossessed, to help them ease off the brakes and practice random acts of moving forward, going at the right speed with helpers obeying the traffic signals. Help those we care for to ease off the brakes.

NUGGET FOR TODAY: I will lift my feet off the brakes and practice random acts of moving forward.

PRAYER FOR TODAY: Lord, you told us to go and do, to spread the Good News. Help us to ease off the brakes of comfort, apathy, neutrality, prejudice, or let someone else do it, and accelerate with the flow of traffic to help those in need. Lord, we know the highways and byways are crowded with those who seem to drive aimlessly, who drive with their foot on the brake, who brake for no apparent reason. Let us be aware of how our driving habits may help or hinder another driver. Help us to know when to speed up and when to slow down, but most of all Lord, give us a spirit of moving ahead, being confident that You can help us ease off the brake and navigate traffic when the time is right...

Wake Up!

Verse for Today: Luke 15:24

For this son of mine who was dead and is alive again; he was lost and is found. So they began to celebrate.

This selection from the familiar parable of the *Prodigal Son* is also among the parables about things that were lost—in this case, the lost son. The father in the story is rejoicing about the return of his son who demanded his inheritance, went to the city and wasted it on riotous, reckless (prodigal) living. When the son's money was gone, the son fell to the low state of eating among the hogs (unclean animals).

The son woke up, came to his senses; he realized his error, realized the blessings of home, so he set out for home. Meanwhile, the father who considered him dead, grieved over his leaving home. Understandably, when the father saw the son coming toward home in the distance, the father rejoiced and held a welcoming party for the son's return.

The son woke up; he came alive. How can helpers help those we serve come alive? Many have wasted their earnings, inheritance, and their best chances on reckless living. They seem lost. Many are as the Prodigal Son in our story, so low in spirit that they can't imagine being up. Eating "slop" and leftovers among animals is a low point of despair, loneliness, or depression, and disappointment over broken relationships and what could have been. Sadly, many may not be as fortunate as the Prodigal Son. Even if they come to their senses, they can't always go home.

Yes, we know that people have the tendency to make wrong choices. But do they have to live with the consequences the rest of their lives? Is someone perhaps a mother, estranged wife or husband, sister, brother, friend just waiting to put on a welcome home feast, waiting to put on the robe of forgiveness, the sandals of rejoicing, the ring of love and commitment? Yes, some may have relationships like the older son who was annoyed that such a fuss was being made over his brother's return. But, it's worth the try. Help people to return to the waiting, welcoming arms of loved ones who have been waiting to say: "You were dead, but now you're alive, you were lost but now you're found. Wake up, come home."

Nugget for Today: Today, I will rejoice over the return of a wayward son or daughter.

Prayer for Today: Dear Loving Father, You are just like the father in the story. You grieve when we stray, find our pleasures in the world, destroy our inheritance, and partake in riotous living. You let us stray, come to our senses, and realize that our Father's house is always one we can return to. We thank You that You see us coming in the distance and shout for joy, planning a welcoming feast. We know that others might resent our returning home, but help them to realize how much it grieves You over one lost person, one lost sheep. We take comfort in knowing we can always come home and the table will be set. You always leave the light on for us...

101 Helps for Helpers

More than Enough

VERSE FOR TODAY: 1 Timothy 1:14

The grace of our Lord was poured out on me abundantly, along with the faith and love that are in Christ Jesus.

GRACE, GRACE, AND more grace. "**Abundant**" refers to more than enough. Add the adjective exceedingly and the phrase as in some translations becomes overflowing, beyond measure, infinite, more than enough, plus some.

Grace—undeserved, unearned, unfathomable is what God provides. The faith and hope of Jesus should lead us to say glory to God—Jehovah Jireh—the One who provides. The One who not only provides our daily bread, but the spread with all the trimmings, from the appetizer to the dessert; the one who forgives our debts; the Lord who is a Shepherd to His sheep; the One who casts all our sins into the sea.

As humans, we can predict, but we cannot say with any certainty what tomorrow will bring. But we can rest assured as according to the *New Revised Standard Version* of our text, "the grace of our Lord **overflowed** for me." Overflowing-that's a cup that runneth over, that's abundance, that's amazing grace-grace that doesn't count wrongs, grace enough to go around to everybody.

Americans are truly blessed. Even our poorest have more than many. In my travels to Ghana, Sierra Leone, and Liberia, West Africa, I was saddened over the poverty I saw—but even more touched by the spirit of the people—happiness not despair was on their faces, exuberant singing and worshiping in their spirits. Pity on us who have so much but find so little to sing or rejoice about. Even with the more and more, in our abundance we continue to covet what another has; we seem to never have enough. We worship plenty, and are driven to excess. We waste more than others have or ever expect to have. We don't appreciate the meaning of grace—anything that is unearned, unmerited. We discount its value if it is free. We embrace abundant living even to our detriment—excess, indebtedness, stress, keeping up with others—we even resort to unethical behavior to achieve man-made abundance. In the end, we will need God's abundant grace to get us out of our man-made messes.

As helpers and caregivers, let us help people find the joy in the little things, to be confident that tomorrow will bring its abundance if they just trust in Jehovah-Jireh, the Lord who provides. Help them to understand that having things is not as important as having security in the God whose grace is freely given, enough to go around to everyone with some left over.

NUGGET FOR TODAY: Today I will live in the abundant grace of our Lord.

PRAYER FOR TODAY: Dear Lord of More than Enough. Yes, Your grace is sufficient, but more than that it is exceedingly beyond measure. We cannot even imagine what You have in store for us if we but have faith and love, which are in Christ Jesus. Lord, sometimes we are like the rest of the world. The more we have the more we want. Help us to understand that happiness cannot be found in things. Help us to rejoice in the opportunity to help others, to provide for others through Christ's example, and to find comfort in knowing about Your more-than-enough-plus-some grace. Thank You for Your more than enough blessings...

Simple Addiction

VERSE FOR TODAY: Psalm 34:1

I will extol [bless] the LORD at all times; his praise will always be on my lips.

ADDICTION YOU SAY? Well David shows us examples of simple addiction—addiction to God. King David was the ultimate praiser. The Psalms are full of praise, exhortation, and worship of God. It's as if David couldn't get enough of his Shepherd, his Present Help in time of need. I can picture him as he shouted. "Great is the LORD and greatly to be praised" (Psalm 48:1 NKJV).

Psalm 63 illuminates David's praise in this way: O God, you are my God, earnestly will I seek you. My soul thirsts for you, my body longs for you…(Verse 1). These words would probably sum up any type of addiction, a constant longing, yearning for something that binds the user to the addicted thing, substance, or act.

David had a routine of praising God, meditating on God-morning and evening. David couldn't wait for his "fix", next high, or next dose of his God. Through trials and troubles, David sought God. Through good times David was high with praise. In his depression, David cried out. His prescription for all his ailments was God. In moments of elation, David danced with all his might. In times of escape, David sought refuge in the secret place of the Most High (Psalm 91:1). In the times of calm, David basked in the Majesty of God.

Can we help those we serve become addicted to the God of Creation, the God who has everything under control because He is sovereign? Can we help them find refuge under God's mighty wings of protection? Can we help them develop a routine of praising God no matter what—good times, bad times, hopeless times, times of despair, times of not knowing what to do next? Can we help them find comfort in the many praise hymns and Psalms? Can we help them to find daily ways to get "high" on God? Let's begin to give them daily doses of the One who heals all pains, releases captives from all manner of worldly addictions, to find an addiction that need not be treated by counseling or medication. Can we help them find a support group that strengthens each other in overcoming worldly addictions by focusing on the God who alone can cure their longings?

NUGGET FOR TODAY: **Today I will become addicted to the God of my salvation.**

PRAYER FOR TODAY: Dear Lord, in You alone can one's longings, urges, pain, or self-destructive behavior be cured. In You alone can one find ultimate satisfaction. In You alone can one get the will to throw away the pills, the bottle, the substances, eliminate the habit forever. No worry about falling off the wagon or backsliding with You. May our knowing You as the ultimate Healer translate to those we serve. May we find strength in overcoming any sort of temptation toward worldly addictions. May we turn to You to help us deal with the cares of the day. But, most of all dear Lord, may we help those we serve become addicted to You—simple addiction, the first step in healing wounds, throwing away the crutches, practicing positive behavior, experiencing wholeness...

Interest Free Accounts

VERSE FOR TODAY: Acts 2:21

And everyone who calls on the name of the Lord will be saved.

As FAR BACK as I can remember, my family taught the importance of saving. Regardless of how little we earned or had, we were instructed to give to the church, and put something aside for a "rainy day." Saving has grown to an all-consuming passion for many as they try to maximize what they can put aside by investing, watching interest rates, keeping abreast of trends, juggling money between accounts. For many this consumes a great deal of thought, time, and money; it can be an obsession. Many with smaller amounts to invest, at least try to take advantage of interest bearing accounts to help their money grow.

A modern trend is making purchases interest free. Retailers have provided longer periods of time before "interest becomes due." Some make offers even into the years ahead. Recent commercials and ads promote no interest till 20xx, years away. But, take heed. It's easy to get caught up in the frenzy of this trend—buying what you don't need or can't afford, with money you don't have, buying "on time," as we described it in Georgia. Rather, many try to "buy time" for what they actually can't afford. The irony is, when the final due date arrives, months or years from now, any unpaid interest accrues from the beginning of the contract. So unless the entire balance is paid off by the due date, all the interest becomes due, accumulating more debt than the original amount. By then, that sofa or television doesn't appear so appealing.

God gives us a simple plan about saving—being saved, the ultimate reward for our labors. All who call on His name shall be saved. Simple interest, a simple deposit, no compound interest; you don't even have to read the small print. No formulas or actuarial figures needed, no amortization chart needed to find the monthly installment amounts. No payment coupons to mail in, no on-line banking needed, and most of all no credit check needed. Your account is instantly available, small installments of calling on the Lord, engaging in prayer, praise, and worship are all that's needed to accumulate and draw on our deposits.

Romans 10:13 gives us this same assurance. "Everyone who calls on the name of the Lord shall be saved." All who apply are eligible. Identity theft is impossible, because God has a unique identifier for everyone who calls on His name. You don't have to worry about predatory lending. God does not charge high interest rates or use trickery and deceit. The account is open; just make daily deposits by calling on the Name. This offer is universal. No discriminatory practices involved, no need to even fill out an application.

As helpers, the gift of this simple opportunity to be saved is available. The application simply requires that one confesses with his or her mouth and believes God raised Jesus from the dead. In the real estate industry, "buyer beware" is a common concept. Or if it sounds too good to be true there must be something wrong. Well, in this case, it is too good to be true. No need to contact a lawyer; just sign up to be saved.

NUGGET FOR TODAY: Today I will rest in the assurance that the savings plan provided by God is too good to be true. Thus, I will open my account by simply believing.

PRAYER FOR TODAY: Lord, again You present a simple plan. In our technology-driven societies, we tend to make everything complicated. Help us to see the simplicity of Your plan of salvation and take full advantage of the interest-free offer. We don't have to worry about hidden costs, or gimmicks. We don't have to regularly go online to check our account status. We don't need to be encumbered by watching for monthly statements or calling 24/7 credit lines. Just as with an ATM machine, we have a 24/7 connection to You by simply asking. We also have the assurance that the big print displayed throughout Your Word is all we need to give us the assurance that our intrest-free investment will reap benefits...

No Re-Payment Required

Do not repay anyone evil for evil. Be careful to do what is right in the eyes of everybody. On the contrary: "If your enemy is hungry, feed him; if he is thirsty, give him something to drink. In doing this you will heap burning coals on his head." Do not be overcome by evil, but overcome evil with good."

AFTER SOME HURT or pain caused by another, some people seem to spend the rest of their lives consumed with getting back at the perpetrator. They are bent on revenge; they are determined to not let anyone get away with anything; they are determined to get even.

For some, this simply entails trying to out wit or out scheme others. For all too many, as we have especially seen lately, this getting even is manifested in acts of violence or even death to the perpetrator and innocent victims. The news is replete with spurned lovers stalking and even killing those who broke off relationships. Others are so consumed by revenge that they stopped at nothing to cause harm to the one who wronged them.

Anger management, conflict resolution, restraining orders, and protection orders are common mechanisms in place to help avert one's attempt to get revenge, to help control the angry impulses to harm another, and to get even. Nowadays, people take things into their own hands.

Many bear the scars of being hurt by others. This passage tells us to heap coals [of goodness] on those who hurt us. Vengeance belongs to the Lord. We are instructed to be kind to our enemies by feeding them if they are hungry and giving them something to drink to quench their thirst. Not returning evil with evil brings on the command to do what is morally good and noble. Being consumed by evil toward an avenger brings more harm to the one wronged. A cancerous spirit prevents us from moving on; we can't forgive and thereby experience the freedom of forgiveness. What we harbor internally can manifest itself in both physical and mental illness and a range of maladies in the long run.

Helpers, this is perhaps one of the most important things to try to instill in those we serve. This is an area of great concern. Feelings of vengeance and getting back at someone can lead to self-destructive behavior. For all too many, this has led to addictions, incarceration, estrangement, and a life of misery.

Let's help those we help to realize that vengeance is not meant for us. Trying to repay evil with evil only leads to more evil. God rights all wrongs as He sees fit, when He sees fit, in the manner He sees fit. It's not for us to determine what is fitting and just for another, but rather to free ourselves from the bondage of hatred and revenge. Forgiveness is the only way.

NUGGET FOR TODAY: When I think on the evil that someone has done to me, I will let God take care of it.

PRAYER FOR TODAY: Dear God, Righter of all Wrongs, Your Word says that we should not repay evil with evil. Lord, free us from any thing that may compel us to try to take matters into our own hands. Help us to understand that we do more harm to ourselves by trying to get back at others than by leaving everything to You. You sit high and look low. You know when people hurt or harm us or try to put stumbling blocks in our way. Help us to heap coals of goodness, love, and pardon on those who cause us harm. Forgiveness is more to our benefit than harboring the need to repay the evil done to us. We are not required to repay evil for evil. Thank You for this instruction on how to deal with being wronged. Help us to repay evil with good…

Layaway Permitted

VERSE FOR TODAY: Matthew 6:19

Do not store up for yourselves treasures on earth, where moth and rust destroy, and where thieves break in and steal. But store up for yourselves treasures in heaven where moth and rust do not destroy, and where thieves do not break in and steal. For where your treasure is, there your heart will be also.

IN TODAY'S SOCIETY, very few people take advantage of the layaway opportunity. In fact, many retail establishments no longer have layaway plans, where the buyer makes a down payment to hold an item, and makes regular installments until the item is paid off. With the emergence and proliferation of credit cards, accompanied by the desire to "have it now," layaways are not popular options.

Today's younger persons probably have little knowledge of or desire to lay away a purchase, pay on it and not take possession of it for a while. More popular options are charging or "rent to own." These usually amount to spending a great deal more for the item than by paying cash or putting an item in layaway. Delayed gratification is not a popular notion in our society today. As a student and newlywed, I remember laying away school clothes, Christmas gifts, and furnishings. I was thrilled to make the last payment and take the item home.

The words in today's text lead us to reflect on what is important—earthly, temporary treasures or heavenly eternal treasures. Attaining assets and planning for the future, being prepared for the unexpected are important for our earthly lives. But if these become our priority they will lead to our own feelings of self-sufficiency rather than God-dependency.

We are often like the rich man in Luke 12:16-21, whose crops yielded so much that he had to continually build bigger and bigger barns or storehouses for his crops and goods. He finally arrived at the point where he thought he could rest in his possessions with no worry for tomorrow. Unfortunately there would be no tomorrow for this farmer and he wouldn't be taking his treasures with him as he died that very night. Thus, Jesus warned: "So is he who lays up treasure for himself, and is not rich toward God."

We are often obsessed with more and need bigger and better—closets, barns, garages, sheds to store our earthly treasures. Self-storage places and PODS (Portable On Demand Storage) have cropped up all over. We should be reminded that our acquisitions will be left behind when our earthly journey is over. Who will inherit our earthly possessions?—possibly someone with little regard for the labor, energy, and diligence it took to amass them.

Helpers, it is good to lead those we help and ourselves to lay away spiritual treasures in preparation for heavenly things. We often help those who lack even bare necessities. As I think of the plight of slaves who arrived to the American shores under the banner of servitude, they survived by focusing on treasure that they could layaway for the life beyond. They would hardly own or have the ability to store up earthly treasures; so they focused on the visions of heaven: golden slippers, golden waistbands, white robes, items needed to walk the streets of gold. They longed for wings to allow them to fly above the burden and pains of everyday life. Every day they laid away their timber to prepare for a home that neither thieves nor moths could destroy. To be sure, layaway is permitted

NUGGET FOR TODAY: Today, I will focus on heavenly treasures and lay away things that endure for eternity.

PRAYER FOR TODAY: Dear Lord of the Storehouses, help us to realize that our journey here on earth is temporary. No matter what we amass or attain here on earth, it will be left here on earth when our time comes. We won't be able to take a thing nor preside over how our possessions are distributed; thieves and moths are constantly waiting to destroy our earthly possessions. Help us to lay away those things that will count as heavenly things. Help us avoid being self-focused by hoarding things. Help us to share with others what you have provided to us so we will not be condemned for our obsession for more, even more; bigger, even bigger; better, even better things. Help us to be content with having the blessing of basic necessities. Things on earth are temporary; we want to lay away heavenly treasures so that we can experience the joy of walking on streets paved with gold that You promised...

Name Tags

Verse for Today: 1 John 3:1

How great is the love the Father has lavished on us, that we should be called children of God!

How do you want your name to appear on your name tag? This is a question registrars often ask of seminar, conference, meeting, and workshop participants. I have a collection of nametags from my many years of attending events. Why do I keep them? I don't know—actually they look quite tacky hanging on the back of my office door. But, maybe they are a reminder of the places I've been and the wonderful things I've been blessed to experience over the years. Maybe they remind me who I am, lest I forget.

In this epistle, John gives us all the permission to write "Child of God" on our nametags. We are part of God's family, so our names—first names, middle names, and surnames—reflect that we are God's children. This tells who our Father is, our lineage, and the family we belong to. Being God's children gives us certain rights and certain privileges—we can exhibit the nature of our Father, claim our Father's love, and we have permission to be like Him (Verse 2). We have the keys to the kingdom.

Helpers, we can give those we serve the opportunity to wear special nametags. Our clients face many trials, tribulations, and setbacks. Many we help are cut off from their earthly families. Many will never be adopted or taken into earthly families. Many have bad visions of fatherly and motherly love. Many of their families have cast them off. They lack the lavish love that only a Heavenly Father can provide; they lack the assurance that being a child of God can provide. Their nametags are blank.

In the eagerness to experience a love that only God can offer, the world often loves only those who love them. Many become victimized, ostracized, and used by the false notion of love. May we, the helpers, proudly wear the nametag "Child of God," and may we and those we help experience all that belonging to God's family means. John 1:12 further helps us to understand the nature of our names: "Yet to all who received him to those who believed in his name, he gave the right to become children of God-children born not of natural descent, nor of human decision, or a husband's will, but *born of God*." This is a universal Birth Certificate.

NUGGET FOR TODAY: I will proudly wear the nametag "Child of God."

PRAYER FOR TODAY: Dear Heavenly Father, the One who calls us all by name, lavishes love on us, and calls us children, we thank You for the blessing of belonging to the heavenly family. We know there are many things that we can put on our nametags; we know that we can collect many earthly nametags that only represent earthly families, and earthly connections, and earthly activities. Lord, we want to bask in Your love, and be proud of our lineage in You, and love each other as You do. Wearing the nametag "Child of God", does remind us of how we came to be born, and who we are in You, lest we forget…

Over the Rainbow

VERSE FOR TODAY: Genesis 9:12-13

And God said, "This is the sign of the covenant I am making between me and you and every living creature with you, a covenant for all generations to come: I have set my rainbow in the clouds, and it will be a covenant between me and the earth."

THIS SECOND COVENANT shows God's promise never to flood the earth again. When we see a rainbow, we should be reminded that God covenants with His people. Rainbows are intriguing; they often appear unexpectedly after a rain or storm. Whenever I see one, I am reminded that God keeps his promises. In fact, I have a magnet, which says just that. A rainbow is often faint. If you don't look hard, you might miss it. To me a rainbow seems to represent God's outstretched arms. On a couple of occasions I have had the opportunity to see the full arch of a rainbow—no beginning or end. I was mesmerized by its beauty and splendor. The rainbow seemed to be illuminated; the colors were clear, but meshed together in a way that no human artist could capture.

Sometimes, though as in Niagara Falls, rainbows are pretty predictable. It takes both rain (water) and sun to make a rainbow. The mist from the Falls on a sunny day produces rainbows so close you can almost walk under one. Yes, I believe there is a pot of gold at the end, rather a pot of God's love waiting for us to find at the end of a rainbow—the assurance of God's provisions. A pot of God's mercy and steadfastness should be what we think of in the beauty and splendor of the rainbow.

The rhythms of the earth, the seasons, the rising and setting of the sun should remind us of God's constancy and of the Great Creator—Elohim who continues to mystify us by the beauty of all His creations and His promise to human beings. The rainbow is a sign that God keeps His promises even to the ends of time, for in Revelation 4:3 we see a rainbow around the throne of God, another final reminder of God's covenant.

> Rainbow, rainbow
> What a marvel you are
> You serve as a sign…
> **God's covenant to humankind**.

NUGGET FOR TODAY: When I think of a rainbow, I will think of God's love, constancy, and His promises.

PRAYER FOR TODAY: Dear Creator of the Rainbow, what a beautiful reminder to us of Your faithfulness and Your promises. You painted the beautiful rainbow in the sky with majestic colors. You gave it brilliance with Your mighty power. You created the rain and the sun which in combination, produce the beautiful rainbow. After a storm, the sight of a rainbow is a sign of Your love and the splendor that You provide for us mere humans to enjoy. The rainbow after a storm also reminds us that the storms of life don't last always, and there is a "pot of gold" waiting for us when the storm is over. Lord, we thank You for the beauty of the earth and Your promise in Genesis soon after the Creation that the rainbow would be a sign of Your covenant. We even await seeing the rainbow that surrounds Your throne. We thank You that You made provisions for us and Your majesty is compared to no other…

Pass the Salt

Verse for Today: Luke 14:34

Salt is good, but if it loses its saltiness, how can it be made salty again?

As we become more health conscious, one caution is to consume less salt. Salt substitutes abound. Hypertension, heart disease, strokes, and diabetes are taking their toll on millions in our nation and the world. As I eat in the presence of others, I am amazed over the number of diners who reach for the salt shaker before even tasting the food. Just recently I warned my fellow diner as she was reaching for the shaker that the "grits were already very salty."

Salt adds flavor to food and the right amount varies by person. We seldom cook without it. But, what if one day while cooking green beans we pick up the shaker, pour on the white salt crystals, and the salty taste isn't there? How can the salt be made salty again? We'd hurriedly reach for another shaker or box.

In Colossians 4:6, Paul gives another use for salt with the words: "Let your conversation be always full of grace, *seasoned with salt*, so that you may know how to answer everyone." Do tell! –Salty conversations! Well, in this case salt has another application. Salt can describe how we approach one another. It can be used to help us guard our tongue, and produce tasty, wholesome conversation. So, **pass the salt.**

Salt is also used as a preservative. I remember how my family cured meat when I was a child. It was amazing to think that a side of bacon could last a long time just from the effect of the salt. So again, I say **pass the salt.** Use salt to preserve the things of God, so that you will be the "**salt of the earth**" (Matthew 5:13). Reaching for the shaker should help to season our conversations, guide our tongues, and provide wholesome seasoning to our discourses. Reaching for the salt reminds us that "Salt is good" Mark (9:50) as it represents being a true follower of Jesus.

Nugget for Today: I will pass the salt by engaging in graceful, seasoned conversation so that I may know how to answer everyone.

Prayer for Today: Dear Lord, when we think of this message, let us think of You as having the Divine Salt Shaker. You instruct us to pass the salt, season and temper our messages so that we will be the salt of the earth. Lord, let us not lose our saltiness, because it's not possible to become salty again. We pray that we will control the consumption of the type of mined salt that leads to physical ailments and that we will concentrate on the Salt Shaker of Life, You our loving God, and try to guard our tongues and know how to answer everyone. We know that sometimes the first thing we want to say may not be kind. Sprinkle Your grains of love over us so that we will remain salty, kind, full of grace. Lord, help us to **pass the salt** and glorify Your Son as we go through our activities today and always...

Seating Arrangements

VERSE FOR TODAY: Luke 14:8

When someone invites you to a wedding feast, do not take the place of honor, for a person more distinguished than you may have been invited.

UPON ENTERING A banquet or room filled with guests, the first thing people typically do is look for a seat or look to see who's there. They scope the layout, looking for the dais or head table. They try to sit close to the action or close to someone of distinction. Often an early arrival will hold seats for others. Even latecomers look for empty seats up front, the best seats they can find.

At many weddings, civic and social functions, tables are designated as **RESERVED**—for those identified by the host as being special or important. According to this verse, we are cautioned **not** to seek out the best place, but to take a lowly seat or, in other words, take a seat of humility. Then as guests file in, the host may move you to a better seat.

This all has to do with pride. Who do we think we are? What right do we have to take the best seat or seat of honor? As we work with others, there is inspiration in this passage. This bears out in Luke 14:11: "For everyone who exalts himself will be humbled, and he who humbles himself will be exalted." A lowly seat now, does not mean a lowly seat forever. God gives many examples that assure us that those of low status have places of importance in His eyesight and ultimately in His kingdom. God, the host has a special seat for everyone—a seat for the humble, the least, the last to be invited to the table. In fact, for many "persons of importance" their only seat of honor may be at banquets planned by man. God has a way of moving us to the head of the table-one He has reserved for the humble. So, take a seat! Don't worry about sitting up front since God has **RESERVED** a seat for us.

NUGGET FOR TODAY: I will not seek the head table or seat of honor. I will take a seat of humility.

PRAYER FOR TODAY: Dear Lord, Host of **THE** Banquet, please help us to be humble in our doings. When we are invited to a gathering, let us allow those who may be perceived of low status to find the choice seats. Help us to avoid expectations of being at the **RESERVED** tables, but find ones of anonymity and blend in with the crowd. Let us be content to know that as the Host, You may see fit to move us to a better table. You gave so many examples depicting how the humble will be exalted. Lord, we want to be exalted by You, not in the eyes of man. Help us to help those we serve to find their rightful places at the banquet You have prepared for them, realizing that the Great Feast will be in seeing Your face...

M and Ms—Milk and Manna

VERSE FOR TODAY: 1 Corinthians 3:2, Exodus 16:33

I gave you milk, not solid food for you were not yet ready for it.

So Moses said to Aaron, "Take a jar and put an omer of manna in it. Then place it before the LORD to be kept for the generations to come."

GOD PROVIDES THE type of food we need at the time we need it. God has identified and provided the perfect food for every living creature. Man has coined the phrase "food chain." The smaller serve as food for the larger.

For mammals, the food for babies is milk. The mothers produce milk and the babies consume the milk for a period of time. Giving solid food to a newborn can cause serious problems, as their digestive systems are unable to handle it. When they're ready, the babies move on to more "solid food." Animals drink milk for a certain time and are then "weaned." However, humans drink milk all their lives and even drink the milk of other mammals—cows and goats, for example.

Manna. What exactly is manna? Manna was God's way of providing food to the wandering Israelites as they were spiritually immature, not yet ready for solid food of the Promised Land, in the same manner that Paul described the Corinthians. This curious substance, "manna", was tasty and nutritious, was carefully planned by God. I often think that Holy Communion wafers look and taste like manna did. Just as God provided Jesus as the Bread of Life, there is sufficient manna for each person every day. The Israelites were instructed not to save any for the next day. In faith, they had to believe God would send them manna the next day—in fact, He did for 40 long years—sustaining an entire generation with this provision. If they tried to save it, it became rotten.

Paul's reference to milk refers to New Testament believers who were spiritual infants, babes in Christ. They needed to grow teeth to eat the solid food, to grow their faith. As new converts, they were justified but they needed time to mature. But, lest they forget how God fed them, the Israelites were instructed to preserve some manna for future generations—even until today as God provides physical bread and spiritual Bread in Christ Jesus. Our digestive systems are always ready to consume this Holy Bread.

As helpers, we need to be reminded that many of those we help are spiritual babies, on a path to maturity. They need the manna of God (miraculous provision) to survive each day. They need the milk of nurturing, supportive helpers and supportive networks, and caregivers to meet daily challenges. They are on the path to maturity, to making "solid food" choices, to making appropriate decisions and choices, and reaching their goals. Let's help them move on to solid food, made available when they are ready to ingest and digest it, reminding them that the Bread of Life is always available.

NUGGET FOR TODAY: I will feast on the Bread of Life that's been provided to sustain me this day.

PRAYER FOR TODAY: Lord, You are Manna. You provide for us day after day. We never have to go hungry and we never have to thirst because You provided **M and Ms-milk and manna**. Lord, You instruct us to have faith that each day You will provide what we need, and over and over again You do that. We may often wander in the desert like the Israelites did, not understanding Your ways, not wanting to be obedient even after seeing Your miraculous powers at work. Lord, You provided for them back then, and You provide for us still today if we would simply feast on something so simple, yet so nourishing as Your Manna and the Bread of Life. We pray that we will become more spiritually mature, moving from milk to the solid food of faith and trust in You...

Hearing Aids

VERSE FOR TODAY: 1 Kings 19:11, 12

The LORD said: "Go out and stand on the mountain in the presence of the LORD for the LORD is about to pass by." Then a great and powerful wind tore the mountains apart and shattered the rocks before the LORD, but the LORD was not in the wind. After the wind there was an earthquake, but the LORD was not in the earthquake. After the earthquake came a fire, but the LORD was not in the fire. And after the fire came a gentle whisper.

WIND...EARTHQUAKE...FIRE...*WHISPER*....................

In this encounter, we find that Elijah was on the run from God. He had just prayed that he might die after his encounter with Jezebel. This account of God's revealing Himself to Elijah has many implications for us today. We are surrounded by noise, hustle, bustle, and so much going on that we often miss the still, small Voice of God; the "gentle whispers" go unnoticed.

Elijah was seeking God's reassurance so he was looking for a sign. Elijah had called for lightning, for fire, for revival. He was expecting the spectacular. One would think that a mighty wind, an earthquake, a fire would signal God's Presence—His mighty powerful Presence. But, on the contrary, Elijah learned that God does not always appear in the spectacular—at least from our perspective.

We are often looking for the spectacular to represent and reveal God; we want to see it and hear it when it happens— we don't want to miss it.

F-I-R-E-W-O-R-K-S! A-C-T-I-O-N!

That's want we want. We don't want to take time to still ourselves. The gentle, focused stillness requires that we be quiet and open to the Voice.

But, we must focus, lest we miss the Voice. No prescribed hearing aid needed, because the best hearing aids are ears attuned to listen for the less spectacular, the mundane, the ordinary rhythms of life that are punctuated by the miraculous ways that God uses to get our attention and give us a message of assurance.

The everyday lives of helpers are bombarded by numerous demands. Grabbing breakfast or lunch on the go, fighting the stress and noise of traffic, making case plans, documenting case notes, home visits typify our days. When asking for Divine guidance, we may be too busy to hear, too preoccupied with expecting the spectacular. We should attune our hearing aids to listen to the unexpected, still, small Voice. We will hear it if we would just be still.

NUGGET FOR TODAY: **Today I will put on a hearing aid to listen to the "still, small Voice."**

PRAYER FOR TODAY: Lord of the Wind, Earthquake, and Fire, yes You are mighty and powerful. Yes, You can manifest Yourself in lightning, thunder, winds, earthquakes, and fires. But the most spectacular times are times when You reveal Yourself in the quiet stillness when Your Voice is unmistakable, when we must be still and focus and tune in, turn up the hearing aid that comes only when we listen for Your Voice. All too often we may want Your Voice to be muffled by the wind, earthquake, and the fire. Lord, help us to slow down, quiet ourselves, take time to steal away and bask in Your presence, and sense Your reassurance. We don't want to be on the run from You. We don't want to miss it. We want to run to Your Presence, to have Your Spirit to hover over us while we await Your guidance, the gentle whispers, the still small voice…

Jewelry Box

Verse for Today: **Job 28:15-16, 18**

It cannot be bought with the finest gold, nor can its price be weighed in silver. It cannot be bought with the gold of Ophir, with precious onyx or sapphires… the price of wisdom is beyond rubies.

The "it" referred to in this passage is wisdom. Job's treatise on wisdom comes close to Solomon's found in the Proverbs. Without doubt, both writers express the importance of wisdom. But I ask—what jewels can we find in our jewelry boxes? Do we collect "pearls" of wisdom for our jewelry box? Do we seek "golden" treasures and "precious stones" of wisdom? Or do we pride ourselves in the cut, color, clarity, and carats of the physical stones we acquire?

Wisdom comes from our relationship with God. The absence of wisdom leaves a void, one that cannot be filled with earthly treasures. But we spend much time collecting fine jewels and spend much of our resources to attain them. **Gold in Italy, Emeralds in the Bahamas, Diamonds in Belgium, Pearls in China.** The neon signs and shopkeepers beckon us as we travel to exotic places. Merchants bring out bigger and bolder creations to entice us. The signs, tourist coupons, payment plans, and gimmicks lure us in to see the wares and make our purchases. We fill our fingers, ear lobes, wrists, and now many other body parts with all that glitters.

But, Job and Solomon tell us that wisdom is a better status symbol, a better investment, and a better, more cost-effective endeavor—for the price of wisdom is so priceless that no amount of gold can match wisdom's worth. Wisdom can't be purchased, so it is equally available to the rich as well as the poor, regardless of race, class, gender, social status. That's a good message for those we serve, many of whom have very few worldly jewels.

NUGGET FOR TODAY: I will fill my jewelry box with precious pearls, precious stones of wisdom.

PRAYER FOR TODAY: Dear Giver of Wisdom, may we always seek pearls and nuggets of wisdom. We pray that we will seek those things that make us wise, endeavors such as gaining wisdom that are a positive return on investment. We want our status to be based on wisdom and the knowledge that comes from on high. Wisdom is more valuable than rubies, diamonds, precious metals, or jewels. Let us not strive to know as much about color, cut, clarity, carat but may we become knowledgeable about the instructions of Solomon. We pray that the process of all our doing, and all our getting will be focused on getting wisdom…

Divine White Out

Blessed is the man whom God corrects; so do not despise the discipline of the Almighty.

MY FIRST POST-COLLEGE job was as a secretary in a medical clinic for foster children. I had to transcribe notes dictated by the clinic director. My typing skills have never been better than average, which sufficed for term papers and reports. But, having a job that required that I typed, and wanting to turn out perfect clinic notes during my first job, needless to say this was a scary scene. I spent a lot of time starting over. A wastebasket full of balled up paper was often the testament of my work for the day.

I discovered that onionskin paper was easier to erase on or make corrections on, so I always ordered that. The finished product was better, not too many smudges or holes from erasures. Then! Along came White Out™ or "correction fluid," an amazing product—a little dab covered the error, then presto you could type right over the mistake. No more onionskin paper needed. Then, along came self-correcting typewriters, and word processors, and finally the computer.

But the image presented by Job, points to a divine correction, God's White Out. This response comes after Job's friends assume that Job's suffering is a result of sin. Job then expresses happiness over God's chastening—saying that there is a blessing for the one whom God chastens. Job's experience helps humans understand that although God allows both pain and suffering, healing does come. When God allows bad things to happen, it is to make us better. If we just look at the life of Job and the many lessons to be learned about adversity, we would keep a bottle of God's White Out handy.

So, now with computers that allow one to delete, cut, paste, make perfect documents, correction of documents becomes easier. Even with technology,

I am amazed at the small errors or mistakes that I often overlook. Even with having someone else read a document, mistakes may go unnoticed. So some form of white out or correction fluid will be around for a long time, as only Jesus is perfect.

NUGGET FOR TODAY: I will keep the White Out handy and realize that if God corrects me, I should consider it a blessing.

PRAYER FOR TODAY: Dear God, our Divine White Out, we know that even in our best attempts, we fall short of perfection. In our humanity we make mistakes, we misinterpret, misjudge, misunderstand, misquote, misspeak, misdiagnose, mislead. Even in our best intentions, we may cause hurt or harm to another. Even in our best intentions to serve You and follow Your commands, we falter. Lord, just as Job was able to proclaim that a person should see correction as a blessing, we pray that we will embrace that response when we need correction. Man's technology and inventions have come a long way when it comes to correcting mistakes, but there is nothing that can totally erase the mistakes we make except through Christ. We pray that we will learn to rejoice when You see the need to correct and chasten us...

K-NEED Deep

VERSE FOR TODAY: **Ephesians 3:13-15**

I ask you therefore, do not be discouraged because of my sufferings for you, which are your glory. For this reason I kneel before the Father, from whom his whole family in heaven and on earth derives its name.

```
        KNEES
        N
        NEED
        E
        L
        KNEEL, NEED, KNEES
```

THIS COULD BE a word game about finding all possible ways of connecting these words. Saying these words fast three times can also prove to be a tongue twister. But looking at the interconnectedness of the verb KNEEL with two nouns NEED and KNEES can emerge as a pattern for everyday life. NEED IS BOLSTERED BY KNEELING ON ONE'S KNEES, when KNEE-deep in trials, tribulations, troubles—when one is K-NEED-DEEP.

Bowing one's knees appears often in Scripture. A flagrant example of mockery appears in Matthew 27:29 when the Roman soldiers bowed one knee before Jesus and mocked him saying "Hail king of the Jews." What a way to miss the divine meaning of kneeling or bending one's knee before Jesus the Savior.

In contrast to the disrespect of the soldiers, we see how Christ should be exalted in Philippians 2:10, so much so that at the name of Jesus every knee should bow—in honor and respect, not in mockery. Paul tells the Ephesians how he bowed his KNEES and they too can gather strength in the time of tribulation. Being K-NEED deep is realizing we need Divine help, and part of the formula for gaining strength and being filled with the goodness of God is KNEELING. Oh, to be described as "knobby knees" like James who gained this title from constant praying. The more the NEED, the more the KNEELING. But let us also find the NEED to KNEEL in adoration, and thanksgiving for the One to whom every KNEE shall bow and to the One who supplies all of our NEEDS.

Yes, as helpers ourselves, and for many that we help along their journey to wholeness, we often find ourselves *knee deep in all sorts of stuff and situations.* During these times, the only solution is to kneel in prayer before the God who is able to "do immeasurably more than all we ask or imagine, according to his power," (Ephesians 3:20). Kneeling in prayer and asking for guidance is the only way to be aware and live our lives according to God's eternal purposes. Our destiny is set; the road is not easy; but through action, faith, and kneeling in times of k-NEED, we can be able to comprehend "how wide and long and high and deep is the love of Christ …" (Ephesians 3:18).

NUGGET FOR TODAY: Today I will spend time on bowed knees, kneeling and making my needs known to God.

PRAYER FOR TODAY: Dear Lord and Christ, the One to whom every knee shall bow, we humbly come before You on bended knees, kneeling in homage to You, presenting our needs before You. Lord, we know many take the opportunity for prayer lightly, but we want to constantly know that we can place anything at Your feet. We appreciate the opportunity to come before Your Throne of Grace and make our petitions known. We don't need flowery words, or sophisticated phrases. We just need a humble spirit, knees willing to kneel, and faith that You will handle all that we face, and you will supply our needs. We don't need to make a public display; rather we can bow our knees in our secret places, kneeling before You, knowing that You will hear our prayers. We want to have knees that are worn from kneeling, and knowing the only way that we will be able to totally handle our K-needs is by bringing them to You…

MIGHTY WINGS

VERSE FOR TODAY: Psalm 63:7

Because you are my help, I sing in the shadow of your mighty wings.

NOWADAYS, RESTAURANTS AND fast-food places, even the makers of frozen food use all sorts of descriptions for chicken wing flavors such as Buffalo, lemon, teriyaki, all levels of "hot;" and all sizes wings—wing dings, wing-ettes, and probably soon-to-be mighty wings. Some versions of chicken wings appear on most menus-eat in or carry out. These small wings, pale in comparison to the Mighty Wings of God, and other visuals presented in the scriptures. Isaiah gives us a glorious vision of wings: "above him were seraphs, each with six wings," (Isaiah 6:2). These seraphs constantly proclaimed "Holy! Holy! Holy!"

Another vision of wings is found in Psalm 57:1: "I will take refuge in the shadow of your wings, a sense of protection from the storm." Psalm 18:10 gives us this image: "He mounted the cherubim and flew; he soared on the wings of the wind." Psalm 36:7 provides another: "Both high and low among men find refuge in the shadow of your wings." These visuals point to something more than wing-ettes, rather to Mighty Wings.

A more earthly image is presented in Matthew 23:37, an image of tenderness and loving care. When Jesus expresses sorrow for Jerusalem, the Bible paints this picture: "O Jerusalem, ... how often have I longed to gather your children together as a hen gathers her chicks under her wings." I have had the opportunity to see this beautiful presentation in real life. I remember when during a rainstorm I first saw a mother hen spread her wings for her chicks. I thought she was having some kind of seizure as she positioned her wings to cover the chicks. But, her young knew the meaning of this strange posture and they came running.

This special protection, this motherly care gives an image of God's Mighty Wings as being protection, strength, refuge, loving affection, and a defense in the time of storms. It's mind boggling to realize that God's mighty wingspan can gather all of His creations at one time—if we would only go to Him for protection from the winds, rain, storms, uncertainties of life. This image of the Mighty Wings of God is one that helpers can use with those we help, those we try to shelter from the storms, and those needing the shelter of a Mighty God who has a mighty wingspan, Mighty Wings.

NUGGET FOR TODAY: Today, I will gather under the Mighty Wings of God and find protection from the storms of life.

PRAYER FOR TODAY: Dear God, You indeed have Mighty Wings. You spread Your wings of protection over those who seek refuge in You. You surpass any wing-dings or wing-etts that we may find in restaurants or in super market freezers. You present so many images of protection, refuge, and shelter, that assure us we can weather the storms if we would just do as the little chicks, come running when mother hen spreads her wings. We know that You weep over us just as You did over Jerusalem when we fail to heed Your calling, when we seek to find safety and security in everything and everybody but You. Lord, You mourn over us, and You beckon us to come running—may we willingly come to You for refuge, to gather under Your Mighty Wings...

Ripe-Ness

...And, who knows but that you have come to royal position for such a time as this?

IS IT RIPE yet? Growing up in Georgia, we had the glorious option of letting fruit stay on the vine until it was lusciously ripe. We picked it when Big Daddy or Big Mama said it was ripe. They could tell the ripe moment by the color, blush, scent, or feel. They knew when each peach or pear or plum had reached its ripeness. They even had a foolproof method of knowing when watermelons or cantaloupes were ripe. Still today, people use all sorts of techniques such as thumping or smelling when they go to the supermarket to pick a melon that is just ripe.

In our modern day world however, fruit is picked before it is ripe to allow time for packing and shipping to markets—a longer shelf life. In fact, we buy fruit or tomatoes before they ripen so we can keep them longer. Who buys ripe bananas anymore? We buy them green, but we don't eat them green, and often we let them ripen too long when they're only good for banana bread.

Just as with fruit, all creations have a season of **ripe-ness**, which only God can ordain. The orphan, Esther, was guided into young adulthood by her uncle, Mordecai. He orchestrated her development, ascension, and **ripe-ness** into queen hood. God orchestrated her **ripe-ness** into the right timing for His plan. God orchestrated the **ripe** timing for Queen Vashti to rebel, alongside the **ripe** time for Esther's maturity and confidence to exude qualities for queen-hood. God also ordered the **ripe-ness** of the wicked Haman's deeds to surface, and the **ripe-ness** of timing for Esther to boldly approach the king with a request for her people.

God also orchestrated the king's **ripe-ness** to being receptive of Esther's request and to give her what she asked. The **ripe-ness** of the king's inability to sleep that led to a recollection of Mordecai's relating a plot against the king, created the **ripe** time to appoint Mordecai second in command, and ultimately the **ripe** time for saving the lives of the Jewish people.

With those we help, we have to be involved in planting seeds of success that will grow, blossom, and produce fruit that **ripens** in due time. We need to help those we help know when the time is **ripe** for them to move ahead, take control, and declare, "I'm **ripe**, I'm ready, and I'm called for such a time as this."

NUGGET FOR TODAY: I want to be prepared to move when the time is ripe.

PRAYER FOR TODAY: Dear Lord of the Harvest, only You truly know when ripeness occurs. You plant us in places where we are meant to grow. You nurture us with the cooling waters that feed our spirits. You provide the beautiful sunshine and the shining example of Your Son, to provide the Light that guides our growth. You protect us from the rain and the elements and provide good soil for us to anchor our roots. You prune us to make us better and produce more fruit. Now, Lord, we stand ready for the test. We pray that we will recognize when we are ripe, and burst forward in all our blushing, glowing radiance, and be examples of the luscious fruit that You made us to be…

The Yeast Effect

VERSE FOR TODAY: 1 Corinthians 5:6

Your boasting is not good. Don't you know that a little yeast works through the whole batch of dough?

A LITTLE GOES a long way.

"A little dab will do you," says the Vitalis™ commercial.

A little does a lot. Anyone who has ever baked bread or rolls knows that yeast and baking powder make the difference between flat, hard rolls for example, and tasty, fluffy, melt-in your mouth, heavenly-tasting treats.

I think our parents had this passage in mind as they admonished us about the "company we kept." They were concerned over the "yeast effect" of associating with those who had different teachings, ideas, upbringing, and values. They knew how a pinch of bad influence could spread swiftly and profusely, thus weakening their teachings and leading us down an undesired path. So to avoid the "yeast effect" they endeavored to keep us away from the pinch of effect that could override their teachings. A further reminder is found in Galatians 5:9, "A little yeast works through the whole batch of dough"—a reference to false doctrine in this case. Our parents knew best. Before they knew it, little by little their teachings could erode by association—the "yeast effect."

I challenge helpers to use this analogy of leavening in two ways. A little praise, support, positive affirmation goes a long way. A little celebration of each accomplishment goes a long way. A dash of negative talk and condemnation also goes a long way. We also realize that a little backsliding or falling off the wagon can undo years of therapy, counseling, and making progress.

A little self-pity goes a long way
A little self-esteem goes even   further.

A little doubt and dependence go a long way
A little empowerment goes even   further.

A little holding back goes a long way
A little jump-start goes even   further.

Let's take full advantage of the "yeast effect" and help those we serve to rise to greater heights. Use a pinch of "yeast" to infuse those we serve with power, perseverance, confidence, assurance, and expectation.

NUGGET FOR TODAY: I will be aware of the "yeast effect" and sprinkle positive pinches of leavening on all that I do today.

PRAYER FOR TODAY: Dear Lord of the Leavening, Your Word reminds us that a little goes a long way. A little yeast can make a batch of dough palatable and tasty, desirable for eating. Lord, let us use Your yeast to help those we serve rise to their fullest potential. Let us sprinkle a bit of **love** that will help transcend hurt, loneliness, and emptiness, into the lives of so many who have lost hope. Let us sprinkle a bit of **joy** into the lives of those who have little to rejoice about. Let us spread a bit of **kneading** into the lives of those who see only harsh and severe ways of dealing with their issues. Let us spread a bit of **flavoring** into the lives of those who taste the bitterness of life daily. Let us spread a bit of **preservatives** that helps to reinforce and maintain healthy, positive attitudes. Lord, infuse us with the leavening we need to help others; we want to employ the "yeast effect"...

Cracker Jacks

VERSE FOR TODAY: Philippians 3:14

I press on toward the goal to win the prize for which God has called me heavenward in Christ Jesus.

A TREAT THAT has been around for a long time is Cracker Jacks ™. This combination of specially seasoned caramel corn and peanuts is a delight to the taste buds. In addition to the delicious edible contents, there is a prize in every box. Some buy the box for the prize.

You have to search for the best parts—for me, the peanuts are the prize. The picture on the box shows caramel corn with loads of peanuts. When one opens the box, however, the few peanuts have mostly settled to the bottom of the box. Similarly, with the prize, the picture on the box entices us. Over the years the price of a box of Cracker Jacks has risen; the peanuts are fewer; and the prize is less exciting. Further the prize is also toward the bottom of the box. The eater has to eat his or her way to the prize. As a child, I would pour the contents on a napkin, with my eyes on the prize. Usually, I was disappointed.

Now, as an adult, I wonder why they even include the prize? More peanuts would do for me. But, I suspect, tradition and the thrill of the prize keep us coming back for more. What about the prize that Paul is referring to? Now, the prize of life, which leads to a heavenly home, is worth savoring a bite at a time; it's worth running the race for.

As we help others, is the prize worth pressing forward for? For those addicted to gambling, for example, is the prize worth it? The odds of finding that valuable prize of a lifetime in a box of treats are probably the same as buying a handful of lottery tickets, or sitting all day at a slot machine. But, the thrill, the hope of winning the "big one" is what keeps us coming back.

According to Paul, the biggest prize is not tangible, financial or earthly. The prize of salvation is a sure bet for those who fix their eyes on Christ, the ultimate prize for humankind. Let us use the same thrill and hope for heavenly prizes as we do for the prize in the bottom of the box, or the expectation of winning the big jackpot. Let us keep reaching and pressing forward for the heavenly prize.

NUGGET FOR TODAY: I will focus on the heavenly prize by fixing my eyes on Christ.

PRAYER FOR TODAY: Dear God, the Prize of a Lifetime is Yours to give, the prize of a heavenly home. Lord, we often put all our hope in earthly things, trinkets, prizes, and jackpots that can be deceiving, that lead us to become addicted by the picture on the box, or the possibility of hitting the big one, the desire to go from rags to riches, the urge of just one more ticket, one more pull of the lever. Lord, make us aware that our only sure bet is on You, and Your promises. The only way we can press toward the mark is to stay in the race, stay focused, and arm ourselves against those things that distract us. Lord, we pray that we will fix our eyes on Christ and not get distracted or disappointed by the picture on the box or by false promises…

Gift Wrap

Peter answered: "May your money perish with you, because you thought you could buy the gift of God with money."

WE ARE ALL familiar with the sentiment that there are some things that money can't buy— love, health, peace, and happiness. Each human being has been given "gifts"… "having then gifts differing according to the grace given to us, let us use them …" (Romans 12:6).

We put a great deal of time, money, thought, and energy into gifts. Some people begin shopping on December 26th for next year's Christmas gifts. The art of gift-wrapping and gift packaging continues to evolve: gift bows, gift bags, a plethora of options to give our gifts their maximum appeal.

Sometimes the packaging can fool us. I remember a recent bridal shower for a dear friend of mine. Another dear friend sitting at my table won a prize. She had the opportunity to choose from a table full of prizes. She chose one based on the packaging—the name of a prominent store was on the bag, but the contents were drastically different from the packaging.

I also remember pulling names for Christmas when I was in elementary school. Though we had little, our mother always helped us find the best gifts we could with the budget we had. I remember year after year, the person who pulled my name always managed to disappoint me. Sometimes the wrapping was beautiful, but I always braced my self with, "It's the thought that counts." For some, that sentiment doesn't work. People remain mad and refuse to speak with the gift offender for years because they didn't get the gift they were expecting.

Further, many spend years paying for last and past Christmas gifts. Every year, we give and expect bigger and more costly gifts. Christmas shopping now begins in October—and we literally shop till we drop.

But some gifts can't be purchased with our earthly money; and it's an offense to God to think that everything is for sale, no matter how much money we have. When Simon saw how the Apostles' gifts manifested through the Holy Spirit, he wanted to buy this power or gift. His human comprehension could not even fathom the vastness of the manifestation of God he thought could be purchased. He had earthy profits in mind. But, Peter admonished him—this was something money couldn't buy. Yes, today we think we can buy anything, in fact we say everything has a price. Thank God that in His wisdom He made some things available to all, the really important things that man's money can't buy.

Thus, the gift of the helper can't be purchased. Sure, knowledge and skills can be attained through training, discipline, applying theoretical foundations; but the true ability to help and make a difference comes from the Spirit of God intervening in the lives of needy humans in the persons of helpers and caregivers. So, I encourage us to be grateful for the gift of helping others. Let our packaging be worthy of the gift and anointing we offer through service, love, and devotion to professions and callings, and opportunities to care although we may not see tangible, nicely wrapped gifts as rewards for our efforts.

NUGGET FOR TODAY: **It's not the package, but the gift inside that counts. I will focus on those things that money can't buy.**

PRAYER FOR TODAY: Dear God, Giver of every perfect gift, we thank You that there are some things that money can't buy, and we thank you for the greatest gift of all Your Son, Jesus. If that weren't so, many would be left out of the most important gift, the gift of eternal life. Lord, You are so wise to shower us with the gift of helping and we pray that we will never think that that gift is for sale. Let us know that You impart Your Spirit to us daily as a Guide and Comforter, and that there is power in the Gift of the Spirit. Let us hold that gift sacred and seek to know how You would have us use our gifts for those that many would deem unworthy of even a small earthly gift…

Godly Personnel Practices Handbook

Love must be sincere. Hate what is evil; cling to what is good. Be devoted to one another in brotherly love. Honor one another above yourselves. Never be lacking in zeal, but keep your spiritual fervor, serving the Lord. Be joyful in hope, patient in affliction, faithful in prayer. Share with God's people who are in need. Practice hospitality.

SUPPOSE THE FIRST page of the personnel practices handbook you received the first day of orientation for your new job listed one of the first expectations was to: "behave like a Christian." The statement might read: A key element for all employees of this organization is to become aware of all manners of the day-to-day operations. The first major expectation is that all employees *"behave like a Christian."* Obviously this expectation would be in very limited contexts, but let's explore what that means in light of the *New King James* interpretation of this passage.

1.) Let love be without hypocrisy
2.) Abhor what is evil
3.) Cling to what is good
4.) Be kindly affectionate to one another with brotherly love
5.) Do not lag in diligence
6.) Be fervent in spirit-serving the Lord
7.) Rejoice in hope
8.) Be patient in tribulation, continuing, steadfastly in prayer
9.) Distributing to the needs of the saints
10.) Given to hospitality

You might read the first two items, and think okay, that seems doable. But then as you read the list further, would you begin to wonder if you made a mistake in accepting the position? Or, would you say, wow! I've finally landed in a place where I am comfortable? Praise God!

Although in the United States we firmly legislate separation of Church and State, and don't condone religion in the workplace, what would our places of employment be like if we followed the practices laid out for a Christian worker? In other words, I strongly believe we would have less need for diversity/sensitivity training, ethics training, continuing education classes, conflict management training, arbitrators, retreats, respite, civil lawsuits, strikes, bankruptcies, and the like. Our workplaces would be ones that employees would look forward to on Monday mornings, ones in which productivity is high, ones in which people genuinely care about the needs of their co-workers, and ones in which we would care for the community.

As helpers, we cannot impose religion on those we serve, but we can integrate spirituality into our times with clients. Many of those we serve have been beat up by the world and the workplace, so the contents of this Christian worker handbook can become components of the treatment plan. How can we help those we serve to most of all be diligent, to cling to what is good, to be patient in tribulation, and most importantly, to be fervent in prayer?

NUGGET FOR TODAY: **I will utilize the Godly Personnel Practices as part of my job description.**

PRAYER FOR TODAY: Dear Author of the Divine Personnel Practices Handbook, let us be attuned to those things expected as part of the day-to-day operations of our workplaces and our lives. Let us embody love, goodness, kindness, diligence, fervent service, rejoicing, patience, steadfastness, and hospitality. Lord let us engage these so often that they become part of our being and become second nature to us regardless of what those around us are doing. Let us live each day knowing that we should behave in a manner that honors You, and therefore we will guard what we partake in. Help us to be an example to those we serve, and help us to inspire them to ascribe to the things that we also hope to embody: Godly practices...

Espionage

VERSE FOR TODAY: Joshua 2:8

*Before the spies lay down for the night, she went up on the roof and said to them,
"I know that the LORD has given this land to you and that a great fear of you
has fallen on us, so that all who live in the country are melting in fear because of
you."*

RAHAB WAS A Canaanite prostitute, and from our viewpoints, an unlikely
woman to be used in the Lord's plan for Israel. Before leading the Israelites
into the Promised Land, Joshua sent two men to check out the land. Rahab
took a chance. She diverted the men of Jericho who were searching for the
Israelite spies and hid the Israelite spies sent by Joshua. Later, she bargained
with the spies to save her and her family when the Israelites came to overtake
the land. From the scripture, it is obvious that Rahab knew the spies were
working under the direction of the Lord. Her brave actions showed faith in
God, a calculation that earned her a place in the honor roll of faith found in
Hebrews 11:31.

Yes, Rahab took a chance. She provided shelter, food, and safety for the
men of God. She knew about the God that others were living in fear of. She
had heard the stories, and knew the track record of this God. She not only
looked out for herself, but she made the Israelite spies promise to pass by her
house when they were destroying the people and occupying the land. She
engaged in Godly espionage, knowing her efforts would pay off.

As helpers, we need to look beyond one's status in life and realize their
value. Many used by God in the Bible, were unlikely characters, ones most
of us would not put on the call to duty list. It is important that we also
help those we serve have faith like Rahab, to be aware of what's going on
around them, and to advocate for themselves and their families as Rahab did.
Unlikely recruits have potential to be likely servants in God's plan.

NUGGET FOR TODAY: Today, I will look for the good and potential in everyone.

PRAYER FOR TODAY: Dear Lord of the Unlikely, we thank You that You use people like Rahab to carry out Your mission and Your plan. You remind us that everyone has potential to be used by You and that faith is an important quality to rely on when things seem hopeless or we would be destroyed. You also remind us that it is important to plan ahead, make a case for ourselves, and be bold and brave and intentional in asking for Your protection. You remind us that we have many opportunities to act on Your behalf, and entrust the final outcome to You. We want to be listed in the honor roll of faith...

Get in Line

VERSE FOR TODAY: Luke 13:30

Indeed, there are those who are last who will be first, and first who will be last.

IN MOST SOCIETIES, in order to maintain some sort of order in public activities, people are required to get in line—the bank, grocery store, movies, buying tickets, getting good seats, getting to buy "hot" items at Christmas time…We line up or "queue" as in Europe for just about everything. It's a good feeling to be first in line.

Once we secure our places in line, we tend to look around and survey how many fortunates are in front of us and we often relish in how many poor souls are behind us. The length of the line often signals the importance of the event. When we are up front in a long line, we feel fortunate.

Sometimes there are multiple lines like store checkouts or at banks. We constantly monitor to see which line is moving faster. Sometimes, we switch lines only to realize we should have stayed in the line we were in. For me, I always seem to get in the wrong line. Needless to say, waiting in line is not our favorite pastime; it causes stress, consternation, and can even lead to violence if one tries to "cut" in line. We love to be at the head of the line.

The passage for today's meditation gives a different take on positions in line. It is part of the discourse about salvation or the narrow gate. But, what is especially of note, is the turn of events; the last shall be first. In this instance, the line is reversed or "flip-flopped." Many would not be happy with that—sure cause for a riot, especially for those who strive and press to be first at all costs. Some even engage in unethical activities and practices to be first in line. Those who always jockey to be first would never offer that opportunity to those considered the least.

As helpers, this passage offers much hope as we minister to those always considered to be last. If we can help instill hope for those who never experience being first in anything, we can help them find comfort in the fact that being last has some eternal merits in the plan of salvation. This hope helped many Africans in America who were always at the end of the line to survive slavery in America. It should also be a caution for those who must always be first in their minds to consider that one day the line will be "flipped." The last shall be first. Rushing to get in line?

Nugget for Today: I know that one day the last will be first.

Prayer for Today: Dear Lord, yes, You determine our place in line. You know that in man's scheme of things, some always expect to be first, and some use any means necessary to be first. But Lord, You provide the confidence in knowing simply that the last shall be first. You don't care about our earthly positions and status; You don't care about how we jockey for first place; You know that we will always relegate many to the end of the line. You know many feel so important that they even cut in line. Thank You for making it clear that no matter how we "queue" up here on earth, You determine each of our places in line. It's not about who gets there first, but rather by the fact that You have a first place for all of those who call on You…

Temple Worship

Verse for Today: 1 Corinthians 6:19-20

Do you not know that your body is a temple of the Holy Spirit, who is in you, whom you have received from God? You are not your own; you were bought with a price. Therefore honor God with your body.

Next time you eat that extra doughnut, drink one beer too many, drive too fast, talk yourself out of exercising, consider this: our bodies are temples; the Holy Spirit dwells in us. Thus, God dwells in us. Our bodies are not our own to misuse or abuse. Think about that the next time you are tempted to indulge or over-indulge in anything that is not pleasing to God. 1 Corinthians 6:12 states, "Everything is permissible for me, but (emphasis on but) everything is not beneficial." In this current day and age, indulgences abound. This entire passage (Verses 12-20) admonishes us regarding the things that we do to our bodies—the temple of the Most Holy God. Our bodies are members of Christ, should we make them like a harlot? Thus two primal urges— eating and sexual immorality are included in these verses about our earthly temples.

But, what about lack of exercise, daily stress, use of substances, lack of rest, and lack of discipline, all of which affect the body's functioning? Romans 12: 1-2 urges us to "present our bodies as living sacrifices, holy and acceptable to God, our reasonable service." Helpers, the message is simple, treat our bodies as holy places and teach those we serve to do the same. We need to increase our temple worship.

NUGGET FOR TODAY: I will treat my body as the temple of God.

PRAYER FOR TODAY: Dear Loving Creator, thank You that Your Spirit resides in us. We pray that we will let this be a constant reminder and caution in all that we do. Help us to always know that wherever we go, and whatever we do, we take Your Spirit with us. Help us to be mindful that indulgences and over-indulgences are not pleasing to You. Help us to abstain from anything that will desecrate this temple of Your Spirit. Lord, help us to practice mental, physical, and spiritual health every day, and in all that we do. Help us to engage in temple worship…

Fess Up!

Then I acknowledged my sin to you and did not cover up my iniquity. I said, "I will confess my transgressions to the LORD"-and you forgave the guilt of my sin.

MANY KNOW THE story of David's transgression. He lusted for and engaged in sex with Bathsheba, a woman married to Uriah, a commander in David's army. When Bathsheba became pregnant, David arranged for Uriah to be placed on the front lines where he was killed in battle.

David is known for his strong need to ask for forgiveness of this and all his transgressions. This and many Psalms express David's tribulations and triumphs, his sorrows and his joys—but especially his repentance and asking for God's forgiveness. He praised the Lord continually and worshiped with his whole being. David found the Lord to be his strength and his shield (Psalm 28:7), his hiding place (Psalm 32:7). He praised the Lord for His sovereignty (Psalm 97) and His creations (Psalm 8), and His mighty works (Psalm 66). But, when David was in a time of deep despair over his sins with Bathsheba, he knew the only way to move on and claim the greatness of God was to lie prostrate in contrition and "fess up." In doing so, David experienced the freeing, cleansing joy of forgiveness.

As helpers, we serve persons who come with a myriad of infractions against the laws of society and the laws of God. They come with burdens of harms they may have caused to others and with the burdens of things imposed on them. Helping those we serve to "fess up", ask for forgiveness, and to forgive others will help them move forward. As with David, "fessing up" can be a "freeing up" step after "messing up". Fessing up is an important step toward wholeness and healing.

NUGGET FOR TODAY: Today I will "fess up" freeing myself to unload my guilt and move ahead.

PRAYER FOR TODAY: Dear Forgiver of our transgressions, we thank You that You allow us to "fess up." You forgive us and free us from the guilt of our sin. You wash us whiter than snow; You know that there are times that we may lust, make bad decisions, manipulate situations, and cause pain and hurt to others. Lord, we know this is not what You would have us to do, so right now, here today, we "fess up" and ask that You set us free of the bondage of hiding our sins and transgressions, the bondage of failing to forgive others. Like David, we will fall prostrate before You and look for Your healing mercy today. We will praise Your name continually; for we know that You will remember our transgressions no more...

Helping Hands

VERSE FOR TODAY: **Exodus 17:11-13**

As long as Moses held up his hands, the Israelites were winning, but whenever he lowered his hands the Amalekites were winning. When Moses' hands grew tired, they took a stone and put it under him and he sat on it. Aaron and Hur held his hands up—one on one side, one on the other—so that his hands remained steady till sunset. So Joshua overcame the Amalekite army with the sword.

THIS IS ANOTHER interesting account of winning a battle. Moses did his deductive reasoning and realized the secret. Keep your hands up! But no matter how determined the warrior, human limitation prevailed. The laws of the natural world, gravity, took over. Moses' hands became too tired for him to keep them up.

What a difference a few helpers can make. Once they observed what the winning strategy was, Aaron and Hur devised a plan. At this time, Moses was an old man. The young men knew Moses couldn't hold out forever. So, they found a rock for him to sit on to rest his weary feet and legs. Each one held up an arm until the Israelites won the victory.

Holding up Moses' hands represented two things. First, raised hands were an act of worship, praise, and dependency on Jehovah Nissi, the God who fights our battles. Second, with the rod of God in his hand Moses declared: "Today I will stand on the top of the hill with the staff of God in my hands" (Verse 9). Moses was giving a verbal acclamation and a visible indication of the knowledge that the victory would be God's.

Do you have someone to help you win battles? Do you have a trusted friend, co-worker, or companion who can see that you are winning the battle, but realizes your physical strength is failing? Do you have someone to pull up a chair and tell you to sit a spell, and rest your weary feet and legs? Do you have someone to hold up your hands when you become tired and weary?

Are you willing to be an Aaron or Hur to someone else—a client or patient who needs someone to hold up his or her hands during trying times? Or, are you willing to hold up a co-worker's hand, someone who needs relief from the stress and strain of daily living? Can you help those around you keep their hands raised until they are victorious? Raise your hands in worship; raise your voice in praise—knowing that God will grant the victory.

NUGGET FOR TODAY: Today I will hold up someone's hand and I will also be willing to let someone hold up my hands.

PRAYER FOR TODAY: Dear God of Helping Hands, You choose such simple ways to help us do Your work and win Your victories. Lord, You helped Moses to realize the secret to victory was raised hands—a gesture of praise and worship even in the midst of a fierce battle. You gave Moses a staff to raise—a sign that the victory would be Yours. You gave Moses helpers to intercede on his behalf. Help us to be able to discern what You would have us do; help us to hear Your direction in the simple things. We pray that You will send someone to hold up our hands when we get weary. As well, we pray that we will be a willing, helping hand for others...

Return on Investment

VERSE FOR TODAY: Luke 7:50

Jesus said to the woman, "Your faith has saved you; go in peace."

IN RECENT YEARS, businesses, universities, and organizations have come up with various ways to increase productivity and accountability. One term in use is Return on Investment (ROI). In general each department or unit is expected to generate products, savings, or increased yield on the amount allocated to that unit from the general fund. In a university, for example, increasing credit hour dollars or other deliverables could be benchmarks. This process, whatever the name, generates the expectation that some tangible, monetary increase will be the result of the investment allocated to that unit.

The woman referred to in this story is a familiar one. She is known as the woman with the alabaster jar who poured precious, fragrant oil on Jesus. What did this woman invest in order to be saved? Besides being described as a sinful woman—her sin is not specified, her act of devotion to Jesus was condemned by the men present. She followed the rules of hospitality by washing Jesus' feet and providing aromatherapy with the special oil. Her act showed the men's lack of protocol when hosting a guest. Yet, she was looked down on for this selfless act.

Her investment was small—a jar of oil, though expensive, and her tears allowed her to spend precious time with Jesus. Her ROI was invaluable, immeasurable, incalculable, and inconceivable in human terms. She made an investment for all eternity—her return was salvation.

What do helpers receive as a ROI—investment of time, money, talent, self, soul, and sacrifice? Our investment is manifested in the work we are called to do. For we are God's workmanship, created in Christ Jesus to do good works, which God prepared in advance for us to do" (Ephesians 2:10). That affirms our calling. Our investment will be worth it.

Sometimes helpers are the balm in Gilead that helps to soothe and heal the wounds of society. We may be the only sweet fragrance that people ever smell, the aromatherapy that is withheld from the poor and lonely and those considered of little worth. For the helper, the ROI is the satisfaction that in some way we provide the fragrance that leaves a lingering, therapeutic effect on those who otherwise would only experience the stench of a cruel world. For the helper, the scent often lingers once we have left the room because it is the essence of Jesus who soothes our longings.

NUGGET FOR TODAY: Today I will spread the sweet fragrance of God's love to someone who needs it. In turn, that fragrance will be therapeutic for me.

PRAYER FOR TODAY: Dear God of the Fragrance, thank You for examples of women and people who take the time to spread sweet fragrance, to soothe another with acts of hospitality. We pray that we will be able to manifest Your call to be a balm in Gilead, that we will live out Your call to model Jesus by doing great works, that we will receive the greatest ROI of all—the gift of salvation. We pray that we might be able to help others overcome the stench of a cruel world with a kind word, a sweet spirit, and a sweet fragrance. Further, we know that the time we spend at Your feet gives us the sweet fragrance of Your love. What a return...

What will You be Known For?

VERSE FOR TODAY: John 20:24

… But he said to them, "Unless I see the nail marks in his hands and put my finger where the nails were, and put my hand into his side, I will not believe."

DOUBTING THOMAS! THIS discourse earned Thomas the eternal name of "Doubting Thomas." No matter what else Thomas may have done before or after this act, it will not replace his doubting legacy. In fact, earlier in Verse 24: "Now Thomas (called Didymus), one of the Twelve," and the Twin, are other references to Thomas. Very few know of the twin designation.

Peter, known as "the Rock" also goes down in history, very prominently for his three-time denial of Jesus as arrest and crucifixion loomed. Abraham Lincoln will be known as the United States President who freed the slaves. Franklin Delano Roosevelt (FDR), another U.S. President who was paralyzed and confined to a wheelchair, is known <u>not</u> as much for his paralysis, as for crafting the *New Deal*. Yet another U.S. President, Richard Nixon, will forever be associated with Watergate; just as Jimmy Carter's founding of Habitat for Humanity will likely be more remembered than his term as President.

What will you be known for? Jane Addams—known as the founder of Social Work; Dr. Spock—modern-day child psychologist; Dr. Martin Luther King, Jr. —Civil Rights leader; Mother Theresa—humanitarian; Dr. Jonas Salk—discoverer of the polio vaccine, are all part of a long list of persons whose names and contributions are instantly recognized. Will your name be added to the list of pioneers, trailblazers, and dedicated helpers? Will you be described as making a difference in the lives of many? It's not important that you may not have a star of fame; more importantly, it's better to have a good name—to go down in history as serving others with passion, integrity, and sincerity. What will your legacy be? What will you be known for?

Nugget for Today: I want to be known as someone who whose life was dedicated to helping others.

Prayer for Today: Dear Lord, You know us by name. You know what others call us. We pray that we will go down in history as being ones who had a heart for helping others, that we took time to listen, that we took time to give guidance and wise counsel, that we were dedicated to help heal the hurts and pains of others. We pray that our epitaph will show that our names will be associated with doing good deeds, taking the time to care, and sacrificing on behalf of others. We pray that a moment of indecision, or a wrong decision will not overshadow any good work that we do. We don't want to go down in history as Doubting Thomases. We know that if we serve in Your name, we will have a special place in history and eternity...

Think outside the Box

VERSE FOR TODAY: Joshua 6:16

The seventh time around, when the priests sounded the trumpet blast, Joshua commanded the people, "Shout! For the LORD has given you the city!..."

THINK OUTSIDE THE box. In meetings, planning sessions, and retreats, we often hear this phrase. Participants are encouraged and challenged to look for new and different approaches to providing services, addressing problems, creating new products, or enhancing organizational development and effectiveness. Today's thinking outside the box example refers to winning a battle.

Many of us probably learned the song *Joshua fit de battle of Jericho* as children. This familiar Negro Spiritual tells of this miraculous victory. The drill was: for six days they marched around the city of Jericho. On the seventh day the ritual was complete. Seven is a significant number—*7 priests, 7 trumpets, 7 days*. On the simple strategy of marching, blowing the trumpets or ram's horns, and shouting in unison on command, the walls came tumbling down.

The strategy was **simple**. It **simply** required following orders, **simple** obedience, **simple** faith, and **simple** outside the box thinking—a **simple** and crude war strategy to say the least. In each era of wars, the strategies and weaponry become more complex and technical. But throughout the Old Testament we see simple tools of war. David used a slingshot. Moses held up his hands. Gideon used noise and confusion—his people blew the trumpets, and broke pitchers. This confused and scared the enemy who cried out and fled.

In modern times, weapons have progressed from bows and arrows to guns, to cannons, to bombs. Countries are amassing WMDs (weapons of mass destruction), new technology capable of destroying entire communities and masses of people. Countries take pride in the size of their arsenals and use that to intimidate others. Might a few outside the box, ordained by God strategies help countries out wit the enemies?

Helpers may need to be reminded that some well-conceived, outside-the-box strategies may be the best way to help win the war on drugs, poverty, and hopelessness. It is comforting and inspiring to see that over the years, spirituality has become more accepted and included in treatment plans. Using herbs, non-conventional treatment modalities, and traditional healers is being infused into the helping plan. Terms such as homeopathic medicine are now included in the range of helping options. Let's think outside the box as we deal with the complex, yet often **simple** needs of those we serve. For all needs, **simple** solutions when blessed by God will make the difference.

NUGGET FOR TODAY: **Today I will think outside the box.**

PRAYER FOR TODAY: Dear God of Simplicity, again You give us an example of how **simple** tactics can help win the victory. Most of us would probably scoff at such simple strategies that You instructed Your people to follow. Forgive our not taking time to identify simple, effective, God-directed ways to help Your people. Help us to think outside the box. Help us to <u>not</u> be constrained by the traditional, but to seek the unconventional in helping those we serve. Help us to be attuned and obedient to the messages You give us that will make a difference in the lives of others. Help us to be willing to be guided by the **simple** things and reflect on the ways You help Your people win the victories…

Gotcha!

Then the Philistines seized him, gouged out his eyes and took him down to Gaza.

I REMEMBER READING the story of Sampson and Delilah—a famous biblical couple—when I was a child. I remember learning how Sampson's mother followed the instructions to rear him as a special child. For one, his hair (the source of his strength) was never to be cut. Illustrations in children's Bible stories show the handsome, long-haired Sampson. He became known for his physical strength, his ability to crush the dreaded Philistines.

But then, Sampson met Delilah. He saw her; he had to have her. She became a part of the Philistine's plot to conquer Sampson. In their private time together, Delilah asked Sampson to reveal the source of his strength. Reading or hearing this story as a child, after the first time, I added words to the page: "Don't tell her; it's a trick!" Even in my young mind, I thought, "He should have known better."

How could Sampson fall for the same ole trick? After each time of giving deceptive answers, Delilah tied him up and the Philistines pounced on him. Couldn't he tell it was a trick? But Delilah challenged his love for her, and each time he gave in. The fourth time Sampson told her the truth. By then he had lost God's favor. **Gotcha!** The Philistines pounced on him and gouged out his eyes, bringing a sad ending to a special beginning—the happiness of a previously barren mother.

I believe helpers see such stories playing out with many they serve. Clients, patients, and parishioners continue to put themselves at risk. They continue to make the same mistakes. Fueled by their own needs and driven by passion and oftentimes deceived by love, they return to the same setting where someone is waiting to pounce on them and delight in saying, **"Gotcha!"** So often those "**gotcha**" things and persons that they can't seem to escape thwart the gains made through the healing process; the ending seems hopeless. So, helpers let us be determined to help those we serve avoid those "**gotcha**" moments.

Nugget for Today: Today, I will try to avoid "gotcha" people and "gotcha" situations.

Prayer for Today: Dear Lord, how often do we keep making the same mistakes? How often do we keep going back to those persons and activities that are waiting to ensnare us? How often do we know we will be hearing "gotcha" but we keep setting ourselves up? O Loving God, we pray that You will give us strength when we face those moments of temptation. Lord, we pray that we won't play around with or take lightly our gifts and strength and lose Your favor. We thank You for being patient with us. Help us to avoid those situations and actions that are not for our ultimate good and help us to lead those we help to do the same. Help us to not play tricks or tempt fate by being childish and arrogant. Help us to be grateful for our strengths, cherish our successes, and avoid "gotcha" situations...

Till Death Do Us Part

VERSE FOR TODAY: Ruth 1:16-17

But Ruth replied, "Don't urge me to leave you or to turn back from you. Where you go I will go, and where you stay I will stay. Your people will be my people and your God my God. Where you die I will die and there I will be buried."

"TILL DEATH DO us part" is part of the vision and ritual for marriage. At weddings the officiant charges the couple to commit to each other "till parted by death." The couple repeats these words of commitment before all assembled. In this story, however, we find a young widow (Ruth) committing to remain with her widowed mother-in-law (Naomi) till parted by death.

Mother-in-law and daughter-in-law return to Naomi's homeland to begin life anew after losing their husbands. Ruth is not familiar with the laws, customs, God, or practices of Naomi's homeland. But, this story points out two very important roles. In order to survive, both women had to trust each other. Ruth trusted Naomi to teach her the ways of her new home. The older Naomi trusted Ruth to follow her leadings and teachings. Naomi taught Ruth to glean grain needed to make bread. She also taught Ruth how to capture the heart of the wealthy Boaz, all the while being a lady and respecting herself.

In watching Ruth, Boaz noticed her demeanor and determination and ordered extra grain to be left in her path. He also ordered protection for her. This trusting relationship of Naomi and Ruth (mentor/mentee), led to the marriage of Boaz and Ruth. Their offspring became part of the lineage of Jesus. Boaz realized the gem he found in the young widow. He also had the opportunity to redeem his kindred, Naomi.

Helpers, how easy is it for us to mentor others? We can find many lessons in this story. The first one is the importance of teaching young people to respect themselves. Secondly, we can become role models. Ruth learned the ways of her new homeland by observing Naomi. Ruth learned to know Naomi's God by Naomi's actions. Thirdly, we can serve as mentors by teaching others the ropes and making things happen on their behalf. Fourthly, we can serve as cheerleaders by cheering others on to victory. In addition, we can pass on the culture by helping others to know the rules, the regulations, and the protocol of our surroundings. Lastly and importantly, we can rejoice! Naomi rejoiced when Ruth found a husband. Ruth rejoiced in her ability to take care of her mother-in-law! This was a mutually beneficial, till death do us part relationship. Naomi especially rejoiced in the birth of Obed, the father of Jesse, the father of David.

NUGGET FOR TODAY: I will commit to helping young persons by becoming a role model, mentor, cheerleader, and culture bearer for them.

PRAYER FOR TODAY: Lord of Eternity, You gave us a beautiful story and a beautiful picture of commitment and relationships in the lives of Naomi and Ruth. You showed an example of how an older woman—though bitter, helped a younger woman— though saddened—to put aside their pain and help each other survive. We pray that we will be able to mentor someone, and we pray that we will follow the leading of mentors You put in our lives. When things seem bleak, help us to make the best of situations and to also look with faith and hope toward a better day, to become like Naomi, bitter no more...

Memory Joggers

VERSE FOR TODAY: 1 Samuel 17: 34-35

But David said to Saul, "Your servant has been keeping his father's sheep. When a lion or a bear came and carried off a sheep from the flock I went after it, struck it and rescued the sheep from its mouth. When it turned on me, I seized it by its hair, struck it and killed it."

WHEN FACING TRIALS and uncertainties, it's a good thing to remember past successes. The Israelites took stones from the Jordan River—stones of remembrance—and built a memorial to remind them of safely crossing over the Jordan River on dry land, to get to the long-awaited Promised Land (Joshua 4:1-7). Many Old Testament patriarchs built altars as reminders of God's protection and deliverance. Noah built an altar to the LORD (Genesis 8:20). In Genesis 12:7, Abraham built an altar that firmed up God's promises and on many occasions, altars reminded Abraham of his encounters with the Most High God. Jacob built an altar (Genesis 35:1). In Exodus 24:4, Moses built an altar at the foot of the mountain. Gideon, David, Uriah built altars. Even observing Passover serves as such a reminder of how death passed by the homes of the Israelites. In modern history, monuments and museums are erected to serve as memory joggers.

The story of David, the little shepherd boy, killing the Philistine giant Goliath, is another often-told Bible story. David had no reservations about going against the taunting giant, Goliath. David was annoyed by how this giant held God's people in fear. His memory sprang into action.

David perhaps had three pictures in mind—lion, bear, Goliath. His memory joggers kicked in and his confidence soared. He didn't need Ginkoba or off-the shelf memory boosters. These would-be giants were "as small as gnats" to David when compared to his God. His shepherd boy experience and tools were fit for the job. The spear, slingshot, and stones were all that was needed to slay this bully who relied on his physical stature to taunt others. In 1 Samuel 17:36, David used his memory joggers: "Your servant has killed both the lion and the bear, and this uncircumcised Philistine will be like one of them."

Helpers and caregivers do you collect memory joggers such as thank you notes, or commendations, or good performance evaluations to urge you on when helping and caring for others? Do you use past successes as fuel for new ones? Do you use memory joggers of how you overcame difficulties to boost your confidence when new challenges arise? Can you set up altars to attest to the faithfulness of God along your journey as a helper and a caregiver?

Can you help those you help to boost their confidence? Can you help them collect stones of remembrance—memory joggers of their past successes to serve as springboards for new ones? Small tokens such as certificates of achievement, notes, award ceremonies, graduations, and even smiley faces can be positive memory joggers. Small successes and accomplishments can lead to bigger ones. Any form of positive affirmations can be used as memory joggers. Keep them coming!

NUGGET FOR TODAY: Today I will collect memory joggers and begin to pass on memory joggers to those I help.

PRAYER FOR TODAY: Dear God of the Past and Present, help us to use memory joggers as we go along each day. Help us to use past successes, past blessings, past hurdles, and past challenges as memory joggers of how You were always with us. Help us to collect stones of remembrance; things that are tangible reminders of Your Goodness and Your Grace and Your Faithfulness. Help us to look on the times when we felt we were about to be consumed by the bear and the lion, by the Goliaths, and using simple war tools such as prayer, faith, and hope saved us. Help us to use the many instances in Your Word of how You saved Your people from being ensnared and consumed as memory joggers of Your on-going guidance, leading, and protection…

Friend In-DEED

VERSE FOR TODAY: 1 Samuel 18:3-4

*And Jonathan made a covenant with David because he loved him as himself.
Jonathan took off the robe he was wearing and gave it to David, along with his
tunic, and even his sword, his bow and his belt.*

JONATHAN WAS THE son of king Saul—the king who became jealous of the
young David—king-to-be. During the times that David was being pursued
by Saul, Jonathan, David's close friend, looked out for David's safety. Later,
Jonathan even betrayed his father by warning David of Saul's intent to harm
him. Jonathan became angered at his father's treatment of David. Jonathan
was a Friend-in-DEED.

In the covenant described in this passage, and borne out through an
enduring friendship, Jonathan, who had a higher position as the king's son,
considered David as an equal. Jonathan exhibited unselfish love by giving
such treasures of armor, sword and bow to his friend. These two remained
steadfast friends. Jonathan's Friend-in-DEEDS extended to occasions of
failing to eat because of his father's actions toward David.

When Jonathan died, David mourned bitterly over his death. David
now had a chance to be a Friend in-DEED. David's Friend-in-DEEDS
extended to Mephibosheth, Jonathan's special needs son who was crippled
as an infant after being dropped by a nurse. David showed kindness by
telling Mephibosheth not to fear. David made this young man a part of his
household, part of his family rather than leaving him alone in an obscure
place to fend for himself.

Everyone needs a Fiend-in-DEED who does Friend-in-DEEDS. Helpers
need trusted friends, confidants, and well-meaning sojourners along the
helping journey. True friends are hard to find, and their help is needed most

in time of NEED. A Friend in the time of NEED, needs a Friend-in-DEED; a Friend-in-DEED helps a Friend-in-NEED.

My dissertation focused on social support networks. Networks can be supportive—providing instrumental help such as money or financial help, and they can be affective—offering advice, counseling, spiritual support, and solace. Everyone needs some of both types of network members. All too often, the networks of those we serve include those who would want to divert a friend from moving ahead and meeting higher goals. Survey your friendships. How many Friends-in-DEED do you have?

NUGGET FOR TODAY: Today I will be a Friend-in-DEED by showing kindness, and support to someone in NEED.

PRAYER FOR TODAY: Dear Friend God, thank You for showing us examples of true friendship. Thank You for those Jonathans who are friends despite position or stature, those willing to run interference and provide help, those willing to look out for our well being, those willing to challenge others on our behalf. Thank You for those Davids who take the time to care for those who could be easily cast aside. Most of all, Friend God, help us to be a friend and to show true friendship, just as You do for us, and so many others who call on Your name. Thank You for being our Friend-in-DEED…

Wise Counsel

VERSE FOR TODAY: 2 Samuel 12:5-7

David burned with anger against the man and said to Nathan, "As surely as the LORD lives the man who did this deserves to die! He must pay for that lamb four times over, because he did such a thing and had no pity." Then Nathan said to David, "You are the man!"

ALONG WITH ADAM and Eve and, Sampson and Delilah, the story of David and Bathsheba comes to mind when we think of Bible couples. David saw Bathsheba, wife of his commander, desired her and set up a scenario to have her. At this time in David's life, he had become king. So, he could command what he wanted.

When thinking of modern-day policies regarding sexual harassment, one factor that comes into account is the relationship of the perpetrator to the victim such as does one have power over another. There was a differential power relationship in this story. David was the king, Uriah was his commander, and Bathsheba was the wife of the commander. David could have his way. This would be considered as sexual harassment. But, David was king; no one would contest him.

The story that Nathan, a trusted counselor and advisor, used to describe a rich man who took a precious ewe lamb from a poor man made David angry. David was that man. Using this story, Nathan made David see the error of his ways. David had his choice of all the women in his kingdom. Why did David have to have the precious "ewe lamb" of Uriah? David was angered and showed his disgust after hearing this story. When confronted with his own sin, David admitted his transgression and spent a lifetime seeking forgiveness.

This story provides many implications for helpers. First, as counselors and advisors to others it is important to give good counsel, to help those we help see their actions and accept the responsibility and consequences of their actions. The child born to David and Bathsheba died at birth. David pleaded, fasted, and prayed on behalf of the sick child; but after the child died, David went back to his normal life, saying, "Can I bring him back" (2 Samuel 12:23)? Secondly, we should never use our position, our status, or our power to fulfill our wants or take advantage of others. Thirdly, it is best to admit our wrongs, ask for forgiveness and try to avoid the same transgression again.

NUGGET FOR TODAY: **I will not use my power, status, or position to take advantage of others.**

PRAYER FOR TODAY: Dear Lord who rights all wrongs, we pray that we will be mindful of our actions and how they may harm others. Help us to be mindful of the delicate "ewe lambs" we encounter along the way. Help us to seek and adhere to wise counsel. Help us to understand how You send others along the way to call us into account for our actions. Help us see different viewpoints or to see the true impacts of our actions. Help us to give wise counsel when warranted and not back down because of someone else's status, position, or power...

Strategic Planning

VERSE FOR TODAY: Nehemiah 2:4-5

The king said to me, "What is it you want?" Then I prayed to the God of heaven, and I answered the king, "If it pleases the king and if your servant has found favor in his sight, let him send me to the city in Judah where my fathers are buried so that I can rebuild it."

OVER THE YEARS I have had opportunities to both participate in and facilitate strategic planning. This process, which typically occurs every 3-5 years, provides an opportunity to review the past, examine the current status of operations, and plan for the future. This is done with the intent to move toward a new or revised mission and vision with new or revised goals, objectives, and strategies.

Nehemiah could have been the perfect strategic planning facilitator. He devised a plan that would hold up to today's Master of Business Administration (MBA) program expectations. After first praying, Nehemiah engaged in three major steps.

- First, as a would-be consultant, he presented his convincing, well-thought-out **proposal** to his boss the king, asking for permission to engage in his task.
- Second, upon his arrival at the work site, Nehemiah surveyed the situation (Nehemiah 2:11), or he conducted a **"needs assessment."** He convened a **"core planning team"**; he inspected the walls, and he made notes, confident that his **vision and mission statement** of rebuilding the walls was the right thing to do.
- Thirdly, Nehemiah conducted a SWOT (Strengths, Weaknesses, Opportunities, and Threats) **analysis.** He assessed the opposition (those detractors and naysayers) and moved ahead with conviction. He drafted his **action plan, identified required activities,** and

developed a **flow chart** that included tasks, and who would do what by when; he identified **outcome measures**, and **timelines**. He also planned to "**roll-out**" the strategy, including a **celebration** upon completion.

Nehemiah realized that adjustments to the plan would be needed; so he developed a **contingency plan**. He also realized that there would be attempts to undermine his work—sometimes by deceit or trickery, even conspiring as, I am sure many executive directors or chief executive officers can attest to when change is underway. But, as any good planner, strategist, or consultant, Nehemiah persevered, completed the wall, assessed the outcome, and celebrated the completion of the task.

As helpers, we often participate in developing action plans or treatment plans for those we help. We have to examine the tasks, needed steps, and needed resources (persons and things); and we need to develop outcome measures—what we want those we serve to achieve before termination of services. May we be **prayerful** like Nehemiah, seeking God's will in all we do. May we be as **diligent** as Nehemiah, staying focused on the task. May we be **flexible** like Nehemiah, making changes and adjustments as needed. May we be **insightful** like Nehemiah, sensing when someone is trying to undermine our work. May we be **resourceful** like Nehemiah, generating alternative solutions. And just as Nehemiah, may we **celebrate** successful outcomes.

Nugget for Today: Today I will engage in strategic planning—I will inspect the walls and spring into action.

Prayer for Today: Dear Master Planner, our God and Lord, thank You that You give us examples of strategic planning. Thank You for the model of Nehemiah, who was burdened by what he heard, who went to You in prayer, and who gained permission to move ahead with his plan. May we be insightful as Nehemiah, inspecting the need, enlisting the helpers, and moving ahead with determination. Lord, we know there will be detractors, distracters, under-miners, and naysayers when they see our moving forward. Help us to <u>not</u> focus on them, to <u>not</u> be distracted by them, but help us to keep our eyes on You, the "Author and Finisher" of our faith. Let us be reminded that faith without works is dead (James 2:14). Let us formulate our mission, grab our tools, and move ahead to Your glory. We know rebuilding the walls will give testimony to Your steadfastness, so we pray for the strength to hang in and hold on until we finish the task. We will then celebrate the victory in Your name and see our planning come to fruition...

Trick or Treat?

Verse for Today: Nehemiah 2:18

I also told them about the gracious hand of my God upon me and what the king had said to me. They replied, "Let us start rebuilding." So they began this good work.

The story of Nehemiah's rebuilding the walls of Jerusalem is replete with several attempts to undermine his work. To counter any obstacles in his way, Nehemiah prayed and trusted God's intervention on behalf of the project. Nehemiah received the blessing of his spiritual King, his God, and of his earthly king, Artaxerxes. So he set about doing his work. No sooner than he had started, three enemies laughed at him, despised him, and accused him of rebelling against the king.

Undeterred, Nehemiah continued with his work. To keep the pressure on, his accusers even threatened him with an attack. What did he do? Nehemiah and the people engaged in spiritual and earthly strategies—they **prayed** and they appointed a **guard**. When the people became discouraged, what did he do? Nehemiah reminded them of their mission and urged them along. When officials tried to take advantage of the poor, what did he do? Nehemiah confronted these crooked persons and demanded that they return the things they had taken.

The story continues… Not to be outdone the detractors tried to distract Nehemiah. He refused their offer to meet in one of the villages (Nehemiah 6:2)—he was on to their trickery. And in Nehemiah 6:9, Nehemiah says, "But I prayed." When they made up untruths, saying Nehemiah wanted to become king, what did he do? He denied the untruths—and yes, he prayed! They even tried to trick Nehemiah into hiding in the temple and breaking the law. Nehemiah realized their motives, and—yes he prayed for justice.

I'm sure we helpers can relate to the obstacles that Nehemiah experienced. Being human, he became angry on occasion, even confronting and rebuking those who were being disobedient and interfering with the progress of the rebuilding. In our work as helpers, we will find all types of people, policies, and positions that try to interrupt our plans and undermine our work to help people rebuild their own walls—their lives. May we use the example of Nehemiah. May we be undeterred. Keep the faith; persevere brick by brick! Assess when an offer is a trick or a treat.

NUGGET FOR TODAY: I will use the model and vision of Nehemiah. I will keep the faith, I will not fuss, just trust.

PRAYER FOR TODAY: Dear Wall Builder, help us to help those we serve rebuild their walls. Many lives are shattered, stones of life are heaped in piles as rubble on the ground. Every day someone steps on the stones, or walks around them. Every day, the wall crumbles even more. We pray, Dear Father, that You will give us the vision, strength, and fortitude of Nehemiah. Lord, we will endeavor to put You first in all we do. Help us to discern "tricks or treats." We ask for Your guidance and wisdom in the situations we face daily. Lord, so many are like the officials in Nehemiah's day; they take advantage of the poor. Help us to challenge injustices, and ward off those who would keep us from the tasks of rebuilding You have given us to do. When we become frustrated or stressed, help us to refuse to fuss; help us to trust...

CEUs

VERSE FOR TODAY: Proverbs 1:5

…let the wise listen and add to their learning, and let the discerning get guidance…

MOST IN THE helping professions require a license to practice in their field. After receiving the initial license or certificate, it is necessary to get CEUs (Continuing Education Units). CEUs are either in the form of taking courses or attending workshops. Failure to obtain the necessary CEUs means losing the right to practice. Likewise, many places of employment require or expect staff to engage in professional development activities to gain new knowledge and attain new skills—they stress lifelong learning. Times change, afflictions and maladies change; new theories emerge; old methods are replaced by new techniques and approaches.

As reflected in our verse for today, the Book of Proverbs, written by Solomon, speaks a lot about knowledge, wisdom, understanding, and instruction. In fact, in the first verses of Chapter 1, the purposes of the Proverbs are listed: *"to know wisdom and instruction, to perceive understanding,"* (Verse 2). Wisdom is personified as a living being—referred to as "her." "Wisdom calls aloud outside. She raises her voice in the opening squares," (Proverbs 1:20). "Wisdom has even built her house and set a table" (Proverbs 9:1-3).

In social work, three words frame our practice: knowledge (know-how), skills (how we utilize our know-how), and values (what we hold to be important). These important concepts are vital for this helping profession. To acquire these is the foundation. Year after year, practitioners must identify, utilize, and develop new practice methods while building on the old. They must find new ways to assess and provide or recommend interventions or treatment. CEUs provide on-going knowledge. But, practice wisdom often is the ingredient that makes the difference. Wisdom is the principle thing, therefore, my fellow helpers, "in all your getting, get wisdom, in all your getting, get understanding" (Proverbs 4:7).

Nugget for Today: Today, I will endeavor to increase my learning.

Prayer for Today: Dear God of Knowledge and Wisdom, You gave us minds, intellect and the capacity to understand. Thank You for allowing us to be involved in lifelong learning. Thank You for opportunities to get CEUs to increase our learning. Thank You that new ways emerge to help those we serve. Thank You that every day there are opportunities to build on our foundation of knowledge by engaging in professional development activities. We pray that we will gain wisdom and find ways to utilize our learnings to help others. We want to listen, and add to our learning, and we want Your guidance as we want to be lifelong learners…

OJT-On the Job Training

VERSE FOR TODAY: 2 Kings 2:9

When they had crossed, Elijah said to Elisha, "Tell me, what can I do for you before I am taken from you?" "Let me inherit a double portion of your spirit," Elisha replied.

WHAT WOULD YOU ask for if you could ask for anything? Riches, wealth, jewels, cars, furs, houses, yachts? Tangible things or health, or happiness—intrinsic things? Would you ask for the wisdom of a wise old acquaintance? Would you ask for beauty, or youth? Or, would you ask like Elisha—would you ask for a double portion of one's spirit? Why such an offer or gift from one about to be taken up to heaven? Why such a request?

Well, OJT (On the Job Training) had paid off for Elisha. OJT occurs when one gets hands-on, applied training and learning while under the tutelage of a master. Known as residency, internships, field placements, student teaching, or apprenticeships, OJT offers an opportunity to learn a trade under the guidance of a learned, skilled teacher. OJT offers the opportunity to try new things under the oversight of a master who knows the job and can help one avoid the mistakes of a novice.

Naomi showed Ruth the ways of her people. Esther learned from her uncle Mordecai. The disciples learned from being with Jesus. Mary learned by sitting at Jesus' feet. Paul provided OJT to Timothy. Elisha learned by observing Elijah. Elisha wanted a double portion of Elijah's spirit, not of his material possessions. Elisha wanted his ministry to be doubly equipped; he had observed a master.

What do you need when helping others? When you have opportunities to learn under the tutelage of a master, will you take full advantage of the OJT? Will you serve as a master, providing training and instruction to others? Will you have the foresight and humility of Elisha to ask for a double portion of one's spirit, determination, and service to sustain your practice?

Nugget for Today: In my OJT, I will focus on attaining spiritual things.

Prayer for Today: Dear Master Teacher, thank You for opportunities to learn on the job. Thank You for those teachers and role models You put in our paths. Thank You that learning never stops. Thank You for the teachings of Your Word, the model of Your Son, and the leadings of the Holy Spirit. Thank You for those whose lives and spirits have touched us; many with the wise things of You. May we not only be partakers and consumers of learning, but may we also pass on to others the things You have imparted to us. Thank You that if we make a mistake, we can always come to You for forgiveness; thank You that You provide new insights into doing things. May we be ever eager to engage in on the job training. And as we are learners, may we also become teachers...

Weigh-In

All a man's ways seem right to him, but the LORD weighs the heart.

WHEN WE THINK of weighing in, pictures of scales enter our minds. Scales of old, with hands and dials are being replaced by modern, digital ones. When we go to the doctor's office, we still step on scales where the nurse moves a weight until it balances with our weight. I always thought those scales in the doctor's office added a pound or two. So, I would *help* the scale by subtracting a pound or two. I would make sure to take off my shoes and sweater just to help the scale get it right.

But, what about spiritual weigh-ins? What additional baggage do we add to the scales of life? This verse hints that people see themselves and their actions as pure, but are they always? God knows the times that we cheated on a test, gave a misleading account of something, embellished our résumés, or intentionally omitted some details. God knows how many times we justified some improper behavior. When it comes to weighing in with God, the spirit in one's heart—noble or deceptive— is what tips the scales.

Examining our motives when we help others should keep us focused on the correct and ethical response or course of action. Doing things out of spite or deception will not only call our values and integrity into question, but also can have devastating consequences for those we serve and ourselves.

It's time to weigh in. I remember when going to the market, there were sometimes accusations that the merchant had his finger on the scales, adding to the weight. We try to make sure our purchases are weighed correctly; do we make sure we weigh our hearts correctly? Are you ready to weigh-in?

NUGGET FOR TODAY: **Today I will weigh in with God. I will examine my heart.**

Prayer for Today: Dear Lord, You always judge us according to our hearts. Lord, help our motives to be pure; help us to do what is right; help us to follow the examples of Christ as we go about our daily work. Help us to ask, "What would Jesus do?" When it comes time to weigh in, we pray that we will be found blameless, not trying to *help* the scales out. We want our testimony to be that we passed the test; the scale was correctly balanced...

Cross Training

VERSE FOR TODAY: Luke 9:23

Then he said to them all: "If anyone would come after me, he must deny himself and take up his cross daily and follow me."

WHAT DO YOU do as part of your daily routine? I try to begin each day with a time of mediation and prayer, then going out for a walk, followed by a cup of coffee, with a bowl of oatmeal during the winter, and cold cereal during the summer. Getting off that pattern can mean my entire day seems out of balance. Oftentimes, however, a phone call, meeting, or a pressing need that rearranges my priorities interrupts that routine.

In this meditation, cross training refers to daily focusing on following God—denying oneself. This routine may be somewhat harder to follow than walking, lifting weights, or working out in the gym. The first expectation of cross training is to deny oneself—to give up those things we can't seem to live without—things, acquisitions, and activities. We are called to take up our cross daily—no exceptions for weekends or holidays—and follow the way of Jesus. This will likely involve hardship and trials, reordering our lives, changing our agendas, and putting our desires second.

Helping and caring for others could be our daily cross. Denying ourselves and unselfishly helping others, embodying the Fruit of the Spirit: *love, joy, peace, longsuffering, kindness, goodness, faithfulness, greatness, self-control* (Galatians 5:22-23) should be part of our daily diets. If we live in this spirit, we won't need to purchase special shoes, or jogging attire, or special equipment. We don't need shoes designed for cross training. We don't need to take pilates, or weight training, or sign up for boot camps. Cross training is good exercise. Our daily routine involves three sets of activities:

Denying,
Taking up the cross,
Following Jesus.
Let's get moving!

NUGGET FOR TODAY: **I will engage in the spiritual exercise of cross training.**

PRAYER FOR TODAY: Dear Father of the Cross Bearer, we pray that today we can develop a special routine. We want to begin every day with "cross training." We want to begin with a time of prayer and meditation with You; we want to get our bodies in good physical condition, we want to eat healthy foods, we want to munch on the Fruit of the Spirit daily, but most of all, we want to practice denying ourselves. Lord, we want to get moving and stay focused by taking up our crosses, and following Jesus...

Laundry Day

VERSE FOR TODAY: **Isaiah 1:18**

"Come now, let us reason together," says the LORD. "Though your sins are like scarlet, they shall be as white as snow..."

WASHDAY HAS CERTAINLY changed. When I was a child, Monday was washday in our neighborhood. We would put water in a big, black cast iron pot along with homemade soap. This soapy cauldron would boil and bubble. With a big paddle, we would stir and beat the clothes until they were clean. Or, we would use some harsh soap on a rub board and scrub away the dirt. After rinsing the clothes in a washtub, we would hand ring and hang the glistening whites and brilliant colors on the line to dry. The whitest whites were the goal of every homemaker. Then some years later, along came Clorox™. Washing became much easier as we would add this magic bleach in the state-of-the art (at the time) agitator/wringer washing machine.

Yes, washing clothes has come a long way. Now, we have all sorts of laundry detergents and additives to accomplish the purpose of our homemade lye soap. Oxy-Clean™ is the new laundry buzzword. Instead of the designated Monday laundry day, we grab a load of clothes, throw it in the washer with detergent and fabric softener, and then throw the clothes in the dryer. We wash while cooking, cleaning, and watching television. Some of us even do laundry daily.

There is one thing that strikes me about this passage. Juxtaposed against the whiteness of snow is the visual of the scarlet. Blood, red wine, and spaghetti sauce—almost impossible to remove even with oxy-clean, bleach, and lye soap—are no task for the Master Spot Remover. This reassuring passage tells us that the stains of our transgressions can become spotless in God's washing machine. He is in control of the wash cycle, no need for additives.

Many live with the scarlet stains of the past—the scarlet of things they have done, or should have done, or things they should not have done, or things that were done to them. Helpers and those we help can take heart that with God, no one is too dirty to become white as snow. A little swirl in the Master's washing machine, using a little grace and mercy as the detergent, and a little love as the fabric softener, God can clean us up. We don't need to use the dryer; we can bask in the **SON** of God's love as we sway in the gentle breeze. It is also reassuring to know that although a day's wear can stain our clean laundry, if we need to re-wash, we can throw the load in again and again.

NUGGET FOR TODAY: I will be confident that God can remove even the most stubborn stain.

PRAYER FOR TODAY: Dear God, our Spot Remover, we thank You for laundry day. We don't need to worry about the wash cycle, the bleach, the detergent, or the fabric softener if we turn our loads over to You. The stains of our day's activities and the stains of our lives have been pre-soaked in Your grace. Your love softens the harsh realities of the spin cycle and Your forgiveness rinses out the entire residue of our transgressions. Thank You that we don't have to worry about sorting the whites and colors; You remove even the deepest scarlet and remove all the spots, regardless of the color or the type of fabric. Every day is a washday; we will give You thanks...

Blueprint Needed

Suppose one of you wants to build a tower. Will he not first sit down and estimate the cost to see if he has enough money to complete it? For if he lays the foundation and is not able to finish it, everyone who sees it will ridicule him, saying, "This fellow began to build and was not able to finish."

HAVE YOU EVER started a project and weren't able to finish it? What things precluded your being able to finish a task? In hindsight, what could have made a difference between success and failure, starting and finishing?

In one of my many drives to out-of-the-way places, I noticed a house where the first floor had been completed for what must have been years. The structure was weatherworn and falling apart. Remnants of building materials littered the property. Every time I passed the would-be house, I wondered why was it never completed? Did the owner change his/her mind; did the owner die? Did the building department put a stop order on the house; did the builder run into problems; or—did the owner simply fail to count the costs and ran out of money?

In this parable, Jesus reminds us to plan ahead. What resources will be needed (people, money, things)? What time frame will lead to completion, and what type of back-up plan needs to be in place? What "what-ifs" need to be outlined? What physical, mental, emotional, and financial costs will be involved? With the rise in bankruptcies, repossessions, and foreclosures, it is a reality that many take on more than they can afford. They tend to live for the moment, until the consequences catch up with them. Adjustable Rate Mortgages (ARMs) became common in the past few years. When the rates became "adjusted" the ability to pay did not catch up. Did they anticipate the costs?

It is important to help those we serve make plans, weigh the costs, forge ahead, and stay the course. A blueprint is needed to guide a construction endeavor. But it is also important to count the costs. Every nail, screw, shingle, board, tile, and gallon of paint must be accounted for. The blueprint is important to help see the big picture, but we must also work with the builder, the architect, and the workers. We must see the short term, step-by-step picture, the big picture, the near future and the distant future. We must keep our calculators handy, and be assured that our buildings will withstand the wind and the rain. We need to add up the costs and weigh the benefits. Our blueprint helps with that. We don't want to be ridiculed. Let's count the costs.

NUGGET FOR TODAY: I will take the time to plan ahead.

PRAYER FOR TODAY: Dear Master Architect, You told us to plan ahead. You believe in orderliness; You guide us to count the costs, to build a firm foundation, and to invest wisely. You tell us not to put our faith in worldly treasures, but to lay up treasures in heaven, so we need to build our foundation by focusing on the eternal. You know that people will ridicule us, so You give examples of dealing with criticism. Lord, in Your Word, You give us so many practical guides for everyday living. We pray that we will keep our blueprint handy and follow Your building instructions as we lay out our plans and as we live our lives daily. Help us to be prepared, to count the costs...

Interruption is Everything

"You see the people crowding against you, his disciples answered, and yet you can ask, 'Who touched my clothes?'"

Celebrities, rock stars, athletes, and film stars experience it all the time. Throngs of people and fans crowd around them, trying to touch them; paparazzi trying to get that all-important front-page photo. Groupies feel that just touching the rich and famous will make them important.

The person in this story, known as the woman with an "issue" of blood, is a woman who had had a flow of blood for **twelve** long years. She had been to all of the doctors, tried everything, spent all her money; but still her bleeding continued. She was an outcast from society, for women who were bleeding were unclean. Nevertheless, she knew about Jesus; she was aware of the healing power of Jesus. She figured if she could just touch the hem of Jesus' garment, she would be healed.

People thronged Jesus wherever he went—people looking for miracles. In this situation Jesus was on his way to heal the sick daughter of Jairus, a layman of high status in the synagogue. As usual a multitude was following him. This woman i-n-t-e-r-r-u-p-t-e-d Jesus' itinerary by touching his clothes. Immediately Jesus knew someone had touched him—a special touch—since he felt power go from him. He looked around to see the cause—the interruption---

Nugget for Today: Interruption is everything.

Prayer for Today: Lord, You don't mind if we interrupt you. We will take time to ponder and reflect on interruptions...

Interruption is Everything!—

Post Interruption

VERSE FOR TODAY: Mark 5:31

You see the people crowding against you, and yet you can ask, "Who touched my clothes?"

VERSE FOR TODAY: Mark 10:47

When he heard that it was Jesus of Nazareth, he began to shout, "Jesus, Son of David, have mercy on me!"

I-N-T-E-R-R-U-P-T-I-O-N CONTINUED... JESUS was on his way to heal the daughter of Jairus— a synagogue ruler, respected in the community—when this woman outcast interrupted his mission. I'm sure Jairus was annoyed by the boldness of this woman. How dare she stop Jesus who was on a more important mission? Who cared about her mission? Why would **she** touch Jesus at a time like this? Her touching Jesus defiled him. Now her touch made Jesus unfit to touch his daughter.

For this outcast-from-society, bleeding-for-twelve-years, spent-her-last-money, down-to-her-last-chance, needing-a-healing-woman-

I-n-t-e-r-r-u-p-t-i-o-n was everything. She touched Jesus' garment. She came face-to-face with Jesus. She found her healing—her faithful interruption freed her from her suffering. She was called "daughter" (Mark 5:34).

On other occasions **I-n-t-e-r-r-u-p-t-i-o-n** was everything.

Blind Bartimaeus, begging for his daily bread interrupted Jesus. Many had passed Bartimaeus by as he sat begging for money. He may have been blind but his hearing was **keen**—he heard Jesus was passing by. Unashamed, Bartimaeus yelled out loudly, "Jesus, Son of David, have mercy on me" (Mark 10: 47).

For this long-time-tired-of-sitting-by-the-wayside-being-passed-by, tired-of-being-blind, tired-of-begging- beggar, all he needed was to hear that Jesus was passing by. Bartimaeus found his healing—his faithful

I-n-t-e-r-r-u-p-t-i-o-n
gave him sight. He became a follower of Jesus (Mark 10:52).

For both of these interrupters, the first response was to ignore the crowd. The disciples were annoyed by Jesus' stopping to interact with the woman. Perhaps they were looking forward to being entertained by Jarius. The bystanders rebuked Baritameus who shouted all the more. They then became encouragers when Jesus **i-n-t-e-r-r-u-p-t-e-d** their rebuke saying, "Call him." Persistence and faith paid off for these and many others bold enough to **I n t e r r u p t** Jesus.

NUGGET FOR TODAY: Interruption is everything.

PRAYER FOR TODAY: Lord, you don't mind if we interrupt you. We will take time to ponder and reflect on interruptions…

Interruption is Everything!—

Jesus Interrupts

VERSE FOR TODAY: John 4:6-7

...and Jesus, tired as he was from the journey, sat down by the well. It was about the sixth hour. When a Samaritan woman came to draw water, Jesus said to her, "Will you give me a drink?"

WE KNOW THIS as the story of the Samaritan woman. This woman was also an outcast. She had had four husbands and was living with her domestic partner, or common-law husband, or significant other. She came to draw water around noon, in the heat of the midday sun. She came to avoid the stares, the whispering, and the ridicule of her fellow women water gatherers. She came for escape; she came for solitude; she came to reflect. She came do perform a daily chore—to get water. She was not expecting an

I-n-t-e-r-r-u-p-t-i-o-n

But there he was this **man**, a **Jew** asking her, a **Samaritan woman**, for water. Didn't he know that Jews and Samaritans, men and women didn't sit down for public chitchat? Couldn't he sense her need to be alone? She was starting to become annoyed; why was he asking her for water?

But, for this woman, Jesus' journey took the direct and more dangerous route. He chose this itinerary to orchestrate their encounter for he knew he "had to go through Samaria" (John 4: 4). He needed to **i n t e r r u p t** her constant thirst for water. The disciples were surprised to find Jesus talking to this woman. But she found out…

I-n-t-e-r-r-u-p-t-i-o-n was everything.

For this seeking-love, unable-to-keep-a-husband, living-with-a-man-out-of-wedlock, searching-for-happiness, tired-of-the insensitivity-of-the-other-women, just-wanting-to-be-alone thirsty woman, she received a drink of water that meant she would never thirst again. She had found a well-spring of Living Water. She became an evangelist and interrupted others by telling them, "I met a man."

Helpers, let us become avid interrupters. Interrupt a conversation that denigrates the poor or the needy. Interrupt a meeting or plans to implement policies or rules that put others at a disadvantage. Interrupt the town meetings, the public hearings, the congressional hearings that threaten to erode the safety and security of innocent humans. Push through the crowds to get the attention of those who can make a difference. Cry with the persistence of Bartimaeus; cry out for the services needed for the blind, sick, poor, lonely, and those who have lost hope. Take time to go to the well, to ponder, to meditate, and to escape the negativity of those who consider helpers to be lesser professionals. You never know what interruption will come your way and ways your thirst will be quenched.

NUGGET FOR TODAY: In this case, Jesus was the interrupter. I will take time today to have chitchat with the One who serves up Living Water.

PRAYER FOR TODAY: Dear Server of Living Water, thank You for interruptions. Thank You for the times You felt the touch of someone tugging at You for a healing and stopped mid-journey to heal. Thank You for the times You just simply asked, "Who touched my clothes?" or as You did with Bartimaeus, "What do You want me to do for You" (John 10:51)? Thank You for the times You intentionally passed through Samarias to sit at the well waiting for someone who had been shunned by others, someone needing love and intimacy; thank You for the times You gave us Living Water, quenching a thirst we could never cure; thank You for allowing us to interrupt Your son Jesus and intercede on behalf of others; but thank You most of all that Jesus interrupts us, stops to chitchat, tells us about our mistakes, forgives us, and allows us to drop our water jars and run and tell the Good News!...

Golden Opportunity

VERSE FOR TODAY: Job 23:10

But he knows the way that I take; when he has tested me, I will come forth as gold.

GOLD—THE MOST DESIRABLE of the precious metals, is a monetary standard, the standard by which wealth is measured. We know that gold has been around for quite some time. The Israelites made an idol in the form of a golden calf while Moses was receiving the Ten Commandments (Exodus 32:4). Golden lamp stands are described in Revelation 1:20. People adorn themselves with gold. Government buildings boast of gold domes; the tombs of the pharaohs, and great works of art display gold in many forms.

Job knew about gold. Once gold is mined, it has to undergo a refinement or "testing" process. Job used this metaphor to assert his innocence to his friend Eliphaz. Job knew he had followed in God's ways. He knew he was experiencing his refinement process. He was confident that this would be a "golden opportunity"; for he was assured that he would come forth as gold. Job knew this was a test, and he had plans to hold up to the *acid test*.

I remember being solicited to buy items of "gold" when I went to Mexico. The vendors wanted to convince the tourists that they were indeed selling gold. They had some chemical that they dropped on the "gold" that foamed to indicate its purity. Well, I didn't fall for it, but a fellow traveler found that the *acid test* was a sham when her item lost its golden appearance a few months after we returned home.

Helpers, how will we handle these golden opportunities? How will we help those going through the refinement process to stand up to the heat? How will we help them hold on to the assurance that what they are experiencing will only be for a season? How will we help them to understand they are "precious?" How will we hold their hands through the furnaces of accusation and guilt? Will we be like Job's friends who held him guilty, or his wife who told him to curse God? Or, will we help them to assert their innocence, their entitlement to better opportunities, and their right to a better day? Will we help them pass the *acid test* and find golden opportunities?

NUGGET FOR TODAY: **I will pass the *acid test*.**

PRAYER FOR TODAY: Dear Creator of All that is Precious, we want to pass the acid test.

Our days are trying,
Our clients and those we care for are crying,
Too many around us are dying,
All too often they resort to "why-ing"
All too often we end up sighing.

But Lord we know every day presents golden opportunities. Help us to stand up to the refinement process. When tested, we want to proclaim like Job, "I shall come forth as gold"...

Changed for Life-The 5 Cs

VERSE FOR TODAY: Isaiah 6:1

In the year that King Uzziah died, I saw the LORD seated on a throne, high and exalted, and the train of his robe filled the temple.

THIS VERSE, WHICH is also used in the meditation entitled "Glory View", is the beginning of Isaiah's commission. King Uzziah, a good king, was also believed to be the cousin of Isaiah. Probably contemplating the loss of his cousin and the end of Uzziah's reign, and sensing his call, the prophet Isaiah went to the temple to seek the Lord. During this time of seeking, Isaiah saw a vision that changed him for life. He saw the Lord in all His glory. He saw the Lord sitting high on a heavenly throne, which represents God's sovereign rule over heaven and earth and His ruler-ship over all earthly kings.

Isaiah also saw the Lord's magnificent garment, a robe that filled an earthly structure— the temple, which also signifies the majesty of God's heavenly dwelling place. After his encounter, which also included six-winged seraphim proclaiming, "Holy, Holy, Holy," doorposts shaking, smoke filling the temple (Isaiah 6:1-4), Isaiah realized his frailties. He cried out, "Woe is me, for I am undone …"(Verse 5).

Isaiah had a Godly encounter and became **convicted** ("I am a man of unclean lips"-Verse 5). He became aware of his **community** ("I live among a people of unclean lips"-Verse 5). He became **cleansed** (a hot coal touched his lips-Verse 7). He became **committed** ("Here am I, send me"-Verse 8); and he was **commissioned** (the Lord gave him a message for the people-Verse 9).

Perhaps many who study the Bible can cite Isaiah's encounter word-for-word. It is a powerful story of how one prophet was changed for life. As helpers, our calling may not have been as dramatic as Isaiah's but nevertheless, we have a strong sense that God has called us to the work of being helpers and caregivers. We are called to examine ourselves, to be 1) *convicted,* 2) to be aware of our *communities*, to be 3) *cleansed* (praying for daily guidance and freedom from any sinful deeds), 4) *committed*, and 5) *commissioned* to carry out the job God has for us as helpers. For many, as with Isaiah, our call to be helpers changed us for life.

NUGGET FOR TODAY: **I want to be convicted, aware of my community, cleansed, committed, and commissioned.**

PRAYER FOR TODAY: Lord of the Heavenly Throne, we thank You that You sit high and look low. We thank You for allowing Isaiah a glimpse of Your Glory—Your mighty throne, the heavenly place where You dwell, the magnificence of Your heavenly garment, the robe that overflows the temple. These visuals that Isaiah describes help us to understand how magnificent You are, that You are the King of Kings and Lord of Lords. We thank You for the example You show us as helpers through Your Son Jesus. We pray that You will continue to convict, cleanse, and commission us to help others. Help us to be aware of the communities You placed us in. We pray that we will continue to be committed to this important calling, that we will cry "woe is me" when we become complacent. We have been changed for life. Send us, we will go…

Blessed Assurance

VERSE FOR TODAY: Jeremiah 29:11

"For I know the plans I have for you, declares the LORD, "plans to prosper you and not to harm you, plans to give you hope and a future."

ONE OF MY favorites, this reassuring verse found in Jeremiah tells us that despite our circumstances, God has not forsaken us. Despite what we are experiencing, we have the blessed assurance that God knows all about it. Despite the worldly assessment of the *state of the union*, we know that there is a Divine set of plans put in place when the God of Yesterday, Today, and Tomorrow set the world on its axis at the beginning of creation.

As with the exiles from Jerusalem who were living in Babylon, the Lord told them to go about life as usual, raising their families, increasing in numbers, and planting their crops. The Lord could see past their current state; He told them to ignore the false prophets because the seventy-year cycle in Babylon would soon take another turn. They would experience prosperity. God had hope and a future planned for them.

This passage is a good anchor for helpers and those we help. We can find comfort in the blessed assurance that God doesn't allow people to be in exile forever. Much like the slaves from Africa who were shackled and brought to America, they were in exile. They left their homes, all that was familiar. They had been royalty—kings and queens in Africa. They faced a bleak future of enslavement and servitude. But they latched on to the blessed assurance presented by visions of the Exodus. They carried on as best as possible, singing the songs of Zion in a strange land. They memorized or book marked Bible passages such as this one when everything seemed hopeless. They never lost hope; they had a future laid out as only God could plan and orchestrate. They knew God had not forgotten them; they had blessed assurance.

Nugget for Today: **I will embrace the blessed assurance of hope and a future.**

Prayer for Today: Dear God of Hope and a Future, thank You that You don't leave us in exile forever. Lord, so often we are burdened by our current circumstances. It's hard to carry on as usual when the weight of the world is upon us. It's hard to see the end of years of bondage. It's hard to keep hope and faith in a future. But You give us the blessed assurance that things won't be bad always. Your Word through the prophet Jeremiah, told the exiles to go about life expecting a future. Your Word through the prophet Jeremiah also told the exiles to ignore the false prophecies of doom. Your Word even told the exiles to pray for the city of their exile (Jeremiah 29:7), for that is how they would find peace. God, thank You that You always have a Master Plan. Thank You for the blessed assurances of hope and a future...

Speed Dial

VERSE FOR TODAY: Psalm 120:1

I call on the LORD in my distress and he answers me.

DON'T LEAVE HOME without it. We'd be lost without it. What would we do without it? It—the telephone? The telephone has gone from a black box with a mouthpiece with an operator to place a call, to a sleek, thin, computerized, multi-purpose marvel. Now, terms such as mobile and landline distinguish the types of phones we use. Digital phones have virtually replaced the old rotary dial phones. At the onset of the use of car phones, only doctors, lawyers, and perceived important people owned the big contraptions. Now, essentially everyone has some type of mobile phone. People use them everywhere, while engaged in some of every type of activity. They talk incessantly, and often distractedly, so much so, that some municipalities have ordinances against using the phone while driving. Yes—this is an important can't-live-without contraption—we think.

But what do we use when we need to call on the Lord? Do you have God on speed dial? I remember a song entitled *"I Got a Telephone in My Bosom."* The enthusiastic singer would point to his or heart and sing about calling on God at any time—*"and I can call Him up anytime."* There would be no busy signal, no being transferred, no being put on hold, no having to leave a voice message, no restriction to call only during office hours, and no having to listen to the Muzak, or pressing numerous buttons, listening to numerous prompts to finally get to the one you <u>weren't</u> trying to speak with. The assurance of this song is you can call God up whenever you need Him; He will answer, and He will answer on the first ring. He knows your distinctive ring tone. He will have an answer before you even hang up the phone, or better yet, He had an answer even before you dialed.

Yes, what a promise. Not only can we as helpers and those we serve and care for call on God anytime, the important reassurance is that He answers. No need for caller ID. God knows you will be ringing before you even pick up the phone; He's not trying to screen calls. And, He has a multi-party line. God can answer several calls at one time, while still giving each caller the individual attention needed. God doesn't try to refer the call to anyone else. He has the answer; just pick up the phone. No need for text messaging; God knows your need and what you want to say before you can even enter the request.

Nugget for Today: I will use the telephone in my bosom to speed dial the One who answers my every call.

Prayer for Today: Dear Phone Operator, thank You for the telephone in our bosoms. Lord, when we are in distress, we will not count on the small, thin contraption in our briefcase, pocket, or purse. Instead, we will make the connection from us to You using the phone that You make available 24/7. What a reassuring thought; we can call on You anytime, anywhere. We don't have to worry about keeping our phone chargers handy if the batteries in our heart are always charged up. You know our distinctive ring; You are waiting to answer. Help us to be wise enough to know when to pull off the road, dial You up, and wait for an answer from You. Thank You that wherever we are, whatever we are doing, we can pick up the phone, put You on speed dial, and receive an instant reply. Thank You that You are always waiting to answer...

Wannabes

Then Agrippa said to Paul, "Do you think that in such a short time you can persuade me to be a Christian?"

LORD, I WANT *to be a Christian* is a song by Delores Lane. Are you familiar with that song? It's a prayer about wanting to follow the ways of Christ. How then do we come to Agrippa's question to Paul? Even in the midst of accusations, while defending himself to Festus, Paul preaches a mini-sermon. He talks about his heavenly conversion; he gives his testimony. He talks about Christ's suffering and resurrection, but most importantly; he talks about the hope of Christ that's available to Jewish people and Gentiles. He poses a question <u>and</u> provides the answer to King Agrippa. "King Agrippa, do you believe the prophets (the question)? I know you do (the answer)," (Verse 27).

What a question. Do you believe? King Agrippa's answer was about time. Can one believe in a short time or long time? Paul was undeterred. Time doesn't matter; do you believe right now? Do you want to be a Christian? Are you a wannabe who will just simply respond to the simple opportunity to believe? Are you a wannabe, but unlike Paul, lack the courage to speak up for your faith? Are you a wannabe stalling for more time, time to ponder the question? Are you a wannabe trying to evade an answer? King Agrippa knew the answer. He knew Paul was preaching truth.

Wannabes can be found in all walks of life. Paul was having an encounter with a king. But, so often we need to confront those we help. We must ask some wannabe questions. Do you wannabe healed? Do you wannabe whole? Do you wannabe free of addiction, free of self-defeating behavior? Do you wannabe employed; do you wannabe in school or in a training program? Do you wannabe a good parent? Do you wannabe re-united with your children?

You can add to the list. Helpers, do you wannabe the one to help those you help get their lives on track, meet their goals, live their dreams? Do you wannabe an instrument, intermediary, intercessor?

Nugget for Today: Lord, I wannabe_____.

Prayer for Today: Dear Lord of the Wannabes, help us today to make our wannabes realities. Lord, we wannabe a help to those we serve and care for. We wannabe an inspiration. We wannabe a role model. We wannabe a coach. We wannabe a facilitator, helping those we serve to put the pieces together. We wannabe true to ourselves and acknowledge our weaknesses. We wannabe strengthened to do the work You called us to do. We wannabe…

Foolproof Diet

VERSE FOR TODAY: Daniel 1:12-13

"Please test your servants for ten days: Give us nothing but vegetables to eat and water to drink. Then compare our appearance with that of the young men who eat the royal food, and treat your servants in accordance with what you see."

THIS BOLD CHALLENGE was given by young Daniel when he was in exile in Babylon. The official in charge of the training of the young men had a regimen that was contrary to Daniel's religious beliefs. Portions of the food served at King Nebuchadnezzar's table had been offered to idols or used in pagan rituals. Daniel knew this would defile him, so he appealed to the officer. The officer was concerned for his job, concerned what the king would say if Daniel and the other exiles were looking unfit and unhealthy.

Daniel knew he had a foolproof diet, one that honored God, and one that honored Daniel's body—the temple of God's Spirit. Daniel in his confidence offered a compromise. He had faith in his foolproof diet, but most importantly in his Foolproof God. And guess what? At the end of the ten days, they (Daniel and his friends) looked healthier and better nourished than any of the young men who ate the royal food (Daniel 1:15).

In this foolproof diet, the food and what Daniel and his friends consumed were important, but the main lessons for dieters are the principles they observed. The main premise of dieting is discipline. Eating the right kinds and amounts of the proper foods, and drinking plenty of water are always components of diets. This discipline was a way of life for the young Daniel.

Helpers, how do we help those we serve maintain the discipline needed for successful living? How do we help them with the right amounts and types of interventions and services provided at the right time to help overcome barriers and obstacles to success? How can we encourage, be undeterred and help those we serve to observe healthy practices? How can we challenge those who would divert them from their goals? As with Daniel, having confidence in a winning strategy, and keeping focused on the goal made known by a Foolproof God are parts of a foolproof diet.

NUGGET FOR TODAY: Today, I will begin a foolproof diet of things that are right for me.

PRAYER FOR TODAY: Lord, of all Diets, thank You for the life of Daniel who stood up to the challenges he faced. He was a stranger in a strange land, but he found ways to adhere to his teachings and principles. He would not be deterred from his life of discipline—his diet, his daily prayers. He found a foolproof diet and he served a Foolproof God who helped him stay focused and disciplined despite those who tried to get him in trouble. Lord, today we pray that we will be like Daniel, that we will stick to what we believe in, that we will speak up for our beliefs, that we will put ourselves on a foolproof diet, but most importantly that we will focus on You, our Foolproof God...

Can You See?

VERSE FOR TODAY: Luke 19:2-4

A man was there by the name of Zacchaeus; he was a chief tax collector and was wealthy. He wanted to see who Jesus was, but being a short man he could not, because of the crowd. So he ran ahead and climbed a sycamore-fig tree to see him, since Jesus was coming that way.

HAVE YOU EVER gone to a parade and couldn't see? I imagine this is how Zacchaeus felt. He knew something was happening—Jesus was passing through. Just as we would want to able to hear and see the bands with their majorettes and flag bearers, to see the floats, to see the cars carrying the officials and queens of a parade, Zacchaeus wanted to see the action.

Last year I had the pleasure of attending some of the early Mardi Gras parades in New Orleans. Heretofore, I had vowed not to be in New Orleans during this time. The crowds and the action seemed too much for me. But, I was there for a meeting of Strengthening the Black Church for the 21St Century (an initiative of the United Methodist Church), and one evening, I looked out of the window of the hotel and I could see one of the floats. People were scrambling for the beads and trinkets being thrown in the street. Yes, before long, I had a front row place, looking down the street for the next float or act. And yes, I was grabbing for beads and trinkets like everyone else.

The excitement of Mardi Gras is one thing, but imagine having a chance to see **JESUS!** Being vertically challenged as we would say today, Zacchaeus couldn't see Jesus. Well, he got creative. He simply climbed a tree. As I watched the Mardi Gras parades, I could see people standing on balconies, steps, statutes, and anything to get a better view. Well, Zacchaeus simply climbed the tree. And, guess what? Not only did he see Jesus, but Jesus also saw Zacchaeus.

Jesus told Zacchaeus to come down from the tree, and Jesus invited himself to Zacchaeus' house (Luke 19:5). That day became a special one for Zacchaeus. The bystanders complained that Jesus was in the company of a sinner. Guess what, Jesus <u>was and is</u> always in the company of sinners—each and every one of them and us. Zacchaeus affirmed his record of giving to the poor and made an assertive response to false accusations. Zacchaeus found a blessing that day. Not only did his tree climbing lead to a better view of Jesus, he received his salvation (Luke 19:9). That was worth the climb!

As helpers, we may need to get a better view. We often need to go out of our way to get the attention of those who can help. We need to climb some trees, shake some branches, extend ourselves, and get out of our comfort zones on behalf of others. We need to attend council meetings and board meetings, and planning meetings; we might even need to make a scene. We need to get a better view of things that impact those we serve. Extending ourselves and climbing some trees may be the only way to see and make a difference in what is truly happening.

NUGGET FOR TODAY: I will climb some trees and shake some branches today. I need to get a better view.

PRAYER FOR TODAY: Dear Lord, Jesus looked Zacchaeus, the tree climber, in the eye and told him to come down from the tree. He received a blessing that day, the greatest blessing of all, salvation. He just wanted to see You, to get a better view of Your Son—he got much more. He learned a lot about You that day because even though he was not liked by his neighbors, You offered him the opportunity to extend hospitality to Your son, Jesus. As helpers, we are often maligned by others because we advocate for the least, and those considered unworthy. We hope to follow Zacchaeus' example by giving to others and holding up to criticism. Lord, let us be willing to climb some trees, get a closer view of You, and allow Jesus to enter our hearts, workplaces, and homes...

What Do You Do?

VERSE FOR TODAY: Psalm 84: 10

Better is one day in your courts than a thousand elsewhere; I would rather be a doorkeeper in the house of my God than to dwell in the tents of the wicked.

BEING A MENIAL servant in the house of God was better to this "usher" than a thousand days spent in the boardrooms and high places. Our work defines us. With virtually every conversation we have with a stranger, one of the first questions is: "What do you do?" Instantly we describe ourselves by our job, or occupation, or status such as retired or stay-at-home parent. The answer usually evokes more conversation if our status seems interesting or intriguing. Or the response can lead to a "that's nice" if seen as common or menial. What do you think the response would be if you answered, "I'm a doorkeeper?"

If you were a doorman at a prestigious hotel or office building who wore a regal uniform, you may get some respect. But, to be a doorkeeper in the house of the Lord? Well, this doorkeeper must have loved his job. Though seemingly of little importance to some, this doorkeeper had the opportunity to welcome worshipers into the Lord's house—His holy temple. To be in the presence of the Lord was obviously a source of humble pride. It was better than being in the highly esteemed places of the world.

So, when asked what do you do, do you proudly proclaim, "I'm a helper?" Are you glad to be entrusted with helping those who need grace and mercy? Are you glad to usher those you help to places of worship, meditation, and solitude? Are you glad to be able to accompany someone to an appointment or advocate on his or her behalf? Do you proudly wear the badge or uniform or demeanor of your profession? Can you say, "A day helping those I serve brings me more joy than a thousand days doing something that is not my calling?" Put on your usher's uniform and help those you serve find their rightful seats.

Nugget for Today: I am glad to be a humble servant to those who need my help.

Prayer for Today: Dear God, our Helper, we thank You for this image. All too often, people look down on the work that helpers do. All too often we look for the high and lofty positions, those that give us extrinsic rewards, rather than thanking You for the opportunity to serve by helping. Sometimes being a helper is not highly thought of, but we would rather be in Your service, serving as a doorkeeper, helping persons find their rightful places. We'd rather help usher persons to a place of comfort and solitude, a place of healing, than choosing a vocation purely based on the pay and prestige. Help us to be grateful doorkeepers, helping to open the doors for those in need…

Multiplier Effect

VERSE FOR TODAY: John 6:11

Jesus then took the loaves, gave thanks, and distributed to those who were seated, as much as they wanted. He did the same with the fish.

EVERY SUNDAY SCHOOL student knows this story—how Jesus took a boy's lunch, five barley loaves (cheap loaves eaten by the poor) and two small fish, and fed a multitude. When it was time for the people in Jesus' audience to eat, there was no food. One disciple, Phillip, surmised it would cost too much to try to buy food for everyone. Another, disciple, Andrew, noticed the boy's lunch, but concluded it wouldn't go far. But with Jesus' divine multiplication—we know the rest of the story. Jesus took the boy's lunch; he gave thanks for it, and he began distributing. Well, not only did everyone get enough to eat, "as much as they wanted", but also twelve baskets with the pieces of the bread were left over (John 6:13). That's the multiplier effect, or simply put, a miracle. **They had more bread left over than they had at the beginning.**

This story has a lot of implications for helpers. First there were two perspectives. Phillip surmised it would cost too much to feed the people. Where have we heard that line of thinking, especially when we look at the cuts made in the U.S. budget for social programs? A few weeks ago, there were reports that the health insurance for children of working parents who still needed help might receive less funding. It would cost too much to insure them. And just this week, the President vetoed the bill for this insurance program.

The other perspective was Andrew's—the five loaves and two fish wouldn't go far. Again, how often have we seen the multiplier effect? How often have we somehow managed to stretch a gift or donation to help more than we thought we could? How often have we looked at the size of the need, like Andrew, without realizing the multiplier effect of our great Jehovah Jireh, Provider God?

We also learn from this feeding of the multitudes that Jesus took time to give thanks. We are reminded to always give thanks for God's provision and to thank those who give of their money and time. Sometimes, just a helping hand makes the difference or eases the burden. Also, the barley bread represented the food of the poor. I often wonder why this boy was the one who thought to bring food? Was he expecting a miracle? Was he expecting to be used for Jesus' work? Was he expecting to linger for a spell? The poor boy gave up his lunch to the Divine Multiplier. His act of giving saved the day. Finally, the beauty in this story is there was more bread at the end of the meal than before. Five loaves not only fed a multitude of men, women, **and** children, "as much as they wanted," there was abundance left over. We also see that Jesus didn't waste the leftovers, he gathered them up. Someone could use them.

NUGGET FOR TODAY: **I believe in the multiplier effect.**

PRAYER FOR TODAY: Dear Lord of the Multitudes, the need is so great, the cupboards are bare. How will we feed the hungry, house the homeless, and help the needy? Lord, we will use this example of the multiplier effect as inspiration to use what we have. We know there have been cutbacks in funding and erosion of the safety net. But, we will trust You to provide the increase. We often feel we are down to our last, that we are out in the field, sitting on the grass, surrounded by the multitudes with nothing to feed them. But we know You can take little and stretch it as needed. Help us to be as willing as the little boy to share what we have, knowing You will use it to Your glory. Help us to guard the leftovers and use them wisely; help us to always give thanks for what You provide for us…

Find a Way!

VERSE FOR TODAY: Mark 2:4

Since they could not get him to Jesus because of the crowd, they made an opening in the roof above Jesus and, after digging through it, lowered the mat the paralyzed man was laying on. When Jesus saw their faith, he said to the paralytic, "Son, your sins are forgiven."

I SAY WE should all have friends like these. This paralyzed man was being brought to Jesus for a healing. His four friends, one on each corner of the mat that held him captive, couldn't get through the crowds, so what did they do? They cut a hole in the roof and let the man down, right in the room where Jesus was. Jesus didn't hesitate to grant forgiveness to this man. I believe Jesus was touched by the faith of the paralyzed man to even trust his friends to undertake this daring and dangerous feat. But, I also believe Jesus was touched by the dedication and determination of these four friends. These friends used ingenuity and creativity to get their friend the physical healing he needed, but their friend received the best bonus of all—he received forgiveness.

The man came in desperation; he left in elation. I can see him jumping for joy even as those around him accused Jesus of blasphemy. Again, we see an example of the healthy begrudging the healing received by the needy. The teachers of the law knew the letter of the law, but they lacked the ability to apply the law to everyday human needs. They would rather that someone missed a blessing if it didn't take place to the letter of the law. We often see how Jesus used compassion to help people in their everyday situations.

There are lessons for helpers in this special story. It is important to have faith and engage dedication and determination along with creativity and ingenuity. These four friends were unswerving in their quest for a healing for their friend. The paralyzed man didn't let fear or uncertainty interfere with his chance to receive healing. The paralyzed man was willing to trust his friends. He came for a healing, but he received an eternal blessing.

It is also important to know that there will always be detractors, those who would use the handbook or manual or procedures or policies to deny services or help. As helpers, we must find a way to circumvent the crowds, find the appropriate place to cut a hole in the roof, and find the right human healer sent to minister to the needy by the Divine Healer. Helpers and caregivers, let's find a way!

Nugget for Today: I will find a way!

Prayer for Today: Dear God, our Divine Way Maker, help us to be willing to find a way. Just as the four friends who thought outside the box to help their friend, instill such determination and creativity in us. Let us not be ashamed of what people might say, but give us the ingenuity and the faith to find positive outcomes for those we serve and care for. We know there will always be those who will criticize the work we do, but let us stop at nothing to help those you send to us. Let us find a way. **AMEN!**

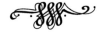

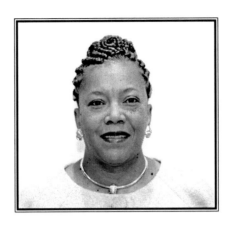

About the Author

DR. LINDA JOHNSON Crowell is an Associate Professor Emeritus, Social Work University of Akron. Dr. Crowell was a social worker for nearly 20 years as well as a research associate before her 11-year career as social work professor. She received a Bachelor of Arts Degree in Psychology from Knoxville College, Knoxville, Tennessee, a Master of Science in Social Administration (Social Work) from Case Western Reserve University and a Doctor of Philosophy in Social Welfare from Case Western Reserve University, Cleveland, Ohio.

She serves Aldersgate United Methodist Church in Warrensville Heights, Ohio as Chairperson of Church Council, leads a Women's Bible Study, and sings in the Vision Choir. She serves the United Methodist Church in several capacities. She is also a member of The Heritage Chorale. She and her husband Henry, a retired Network Administrator reside in Oakwood Village (Cleveland area) Ohio.

Dr. Crowell is the founder of **Help-FULL Source**, a ministry dedicated to providing inspiration and resources for helpers and caregivers.

Printed in the United States
148287LV00005B/24/P